Orthopaedics in Primary Care

Second edition

Professor Andrew J Carr MA ChM FRCS
Nuffield Professor of Orthopaedic Surgery, University of Oxford

Dr William Hamilton FRCP FRCGP
Research Fellow in Primary Care, University of Bristol

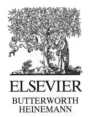

ELSEVIER
BUTTERWORTH
HEINEMANN

EDINBURGH LONDON NEW YORK OXFORD PHILADELPHIA ST LOUIS SYDNEY TORONTO 2005

BUTTERWORTH-HEINEMANN
An imprint of Elsevier Limited

First published 2005
  Reprinted 2005

ISBN 0 7506 8785 1

British Library Cataloguing in Publication Data
A catalogue record for this book is available from the British Library

Library of Congress Cataloguing in Publication Data
A catalogue record for this book is available from the Library of Congress

Notice
Medical knowledge is constantly changing. Standard safety precautions must be followed, but as new research and clinical experience broaden our knowledge, changes in treatment and drug therapy may become necessary or appropriate. Readers are advised to check the most current product information provided by the manufacturer of each drug to be administered to verify the recommended dose, the method and duration of administration, and contraindications. It is the responsibility of the practitioner, relying on experience and knowledge of the patient, to determine dosages and the best treatment for each individual patient. Neither the Publisher nor the author assumes any liability for any injury and/or damage to persons or property arising from this publication.

The Publisher

ELSEVIER your source for books,
journals and multimedia
in the health sciences
www.elsevierhealth.com

Working together to grow
libraries in developing countries
www.elsevier.com | www.bookaid.org | www.sabre.org
ELSEVIER BOOK AID International Sabre Foundation

The
publisher's
policy is to use
**paper manufactured
from sustainable forests**

Printed in China

Contents

List of contributors

Michael K. D. Benson FRC
Consultant Orthopaedic Surgeon, Nuffield Orthopaedic Centre NHS Trust, Oxford

Peter Burge FRCS
Consultant Orthopaedic Surgeon
The Nuffield Orthopaedic Centre, Oxford

Andrew J. Carr, MA ChM FRCS
Nuffield Professor of Orthopaedic Surgery & Head of Department
Nuffield Department of Orthopaedic Surgery, University of Oxford, Oxford

Paul H. Cooke
Consultant Orthopaedic Surgeon, Nuffield Orthopaedic Centre NHS Trust, Oxford

Richard de Steiger MBBS FRACS FAOrth
Director of Arthroplasty, Department of Orthopaedics, Royal Melbourne Hospital, Australia

Jeremy C. T. Fairbank MD FRCS
Consultant Orthopaedic Surgeon, Nuffield Orthopaedic Centre, Oxford

C. L. M. H. Gibbons
Consultant Orthopaedic Surgeon, Nuffield Orthopaedic Centre NHS Trust, Oxford

William Hamilton FRCP FRCGP
Research Fellow in Primary Care, University of Bristol, Bristol

Jane Moser
Orthopaedic Physiotherapy Specialist, Upper Limb Unit, Nuffield Orthopaedic Centre NHS Trust, Oxford

Jonathan Rees MBBS FRCS(Eng) FRCS(Orth)
Clinical Lecturer, Nuffield Department of Orthopaedic Surgery, Nuffield Orthopaedic Centre, Oxford

James Wilson-MacDonald MBCHB FRCS MCH
Consultant Orthopaedic Surgeon, Nuffield Orthopaedic Centre NHS Trust, Oxford

John R. Williams DM FRCS(Orth)
Consultant Orthopaedic Surgeon, Royal Victoria Hospital, Newcastle

Website

Video clips of some of the injection techniques described in Chapter 10 are available at http://evolve. elsevier.com/Carr/orthopaedics/.

The relevant techniques are marked

Preface

Orthopaedic complaints make up a large part of a general practitioner's workload. Few doctors will complete a surgery without at least one patient presenting an orthopaedic problem. Furthermore, as the population ages, the so-called 'degenerative' conditions will continue to increase. As with most conditions, the large majority of orthopaedic complaints are managed entirely in primary care. The aim of this book is to help primary care clinicians to diagnose and treat these complaints, and to assist in identifying the small number who would benefit for referral to a specialist. It has been written to cater both for clinicians in training, and for those who are already in practice.

This is the second edition of this book and draws on the experience gained in preparation of the first. In that edition the initial draft of each chapter was discussed by a group of Oxford general practitioners. This process was in itself educational for the doctors involved, but also led to many revisions. It ensured that the focus remained on problems that would be met in the consulting room. This innovative process was led by Anthony Harnden, an Oxfordshire general practitioner, and the co-editor of the first edition. We have continued in the same spirit with the second edition.

This edition has been fully rewritten and a new chapter added. This poses a range of orthopaedic questions. These are in short answer format, to mimic the Membership of the Royal College of General Practitioners' examination. We have also included video clips of orthopaedic procedures on the accompanying CD. We believe that these will be more instructive than any number of still pictures.

We wish to acknowledge the support and criticism of the following general practitioners, who contributed either to the first edition or to the revision. We are truly in their debt: Martin Agass, Pat Alquist, Julie Anderson, Neil Bryson, Ken Burch, Andy Chivers, Anthony Clarke, Ian Eastwood, Andrew Farmer, Nigel Gilmour, Richard Green, Richard Harrington, Tim Huins, John Humphreys, Peter Isaac, Claudia Jones, Duncan Keeley, Dave Kernick, Tim Lancaster, Veronica McKay, Jane Mortensen, Ben Parker, David Parker, Simon Plint, Michael Robertson, Peter Rose, Dave Russell, Gill Scott, Judy Shakespeare, Simon Street, Tim Wilson, Ken Williamson and Julia Wollond.

Andrew J. Carr
William Hamilton

Chapter 1

Shoulder
Andrew J. Carr

- Shoulder pain is the commonest musculoskeletal complaint after neck and back pain to present to GPs.
- The commonest cause of shoulder pain is subacromial impingement characterized by a painful arc of shoulder movement. It may settle spontaneously but often requires physiotherapy, injection and sometimes surgery.
- Frozen shoulder is also common and is characterized by pain and stiffness. It invariably improves over a 1–3 year period. In the painful phase, physiotherapy is not helpful but injections can be beneficial. Surgery is indicated in resistant cases.
- The posterior and lateral approaches are easier when injecting steroid into the subacromial bursa.
- Two episodes of shoulder dislocation are an indication for surgical stabilization.

PRESENTING SYMPTOMS

The three main complaints of patients with shoulder problems are pain, stiffness and instability. Assessment of the presenting symptoms should differentiate between them. Attempts should be made to determine how these symptoms affect work, life at home and sporting activities. Pain may be present only on activity (usually above-head activity) but can be present at rest or at night.

Pain and stiffness

1. **Is it from the glenohumeral joint?** *If so*:
   the joint pain is present day and night and there is global restriction of movement including rotation (cannot reach behind back or to back of head) *then* analgesics, NSAIDs, then steroid injections (into joint), then refer (physiotherapy only if predominant problem is stiffness).

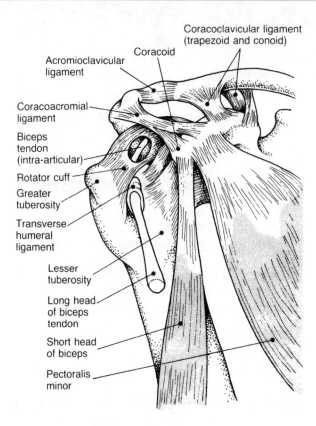

Figure 1.1 Some of the major ligamentous and musculotendinous attachments about the shoulder joint

Table 1.1 Common causes of shoulder pain in different age groups

| Age group | Cause | | |
	Intra–articular	Periarticular	Referred
Childhood (2–10 years)	Instability	Osteochondromas	
Adolescence (10–18 years)	Instability		
Early adulthood (18–30 years)	Instability Acromioclavicular joint sprain	Calcific tendonitis Impingement	Cervical
Adulthood (30–60 years)	Osteochondritis Osteoarthritis Frozen shoulder Inflammatory arthritis	Calcific tendonitis Impingement Rotator cuff tear Bicipital tendonitis	Cervical
Old age (>60 years)	Osteochondritis Osteoarthritis Frozen shoulder Inflammatory arthritis	Impingement Rotator cuff tear	Cervical

2. **Is it from the subacromial space?** *If so:*

the pain is worse on certain movements; movements are restricted in flexion and abduction; rotation with elbow at side is preserved

then analgesics, NSAIDs, physiotherapy, then steroid injections into subacromial space, then refer.

Is it neck or shoulder?
- *Neck*: pain is felt on the side of the neck and over the trapezius.
- *Shoulder*: pain is felt on top of shoulder and over the outer side of the upper arm.

Move the neck and move the shoulder.

Is this your pain?

PHYSICAL EXAMINATION

Inspect

Physical examination should begin with an inspection of the shoulder, particularly looking for areas of swelling or muscle wasting.

Palpate

Palpation can often be useful in determining areas of particular tenderness, such as the subacromial region and the greater tuberosity of the humerus or the acromioclavicular joint.

Move

Assess the range of movement in abduction, flexion and external rotation with the elbow at the side. These movements are measured in degrees. Internal rotation is best assessed and measured by examining how far behind the back the patient can get their hand.

An assessment should be made of power or strength. In addition to grading the strength of abduction and elevation, it is important to assess the strength of internal and external rotation, with the elbow tucked into the side.

Table 1.2   Normal range of movement: shoulder

Flexion	0–170 degrees
Abduction	0–170 degrees
External rotation	0–60 degrees
Internal rotation	Hand to upper lumbar spine

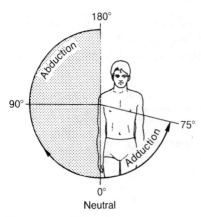

Figure 1.2   Abduction

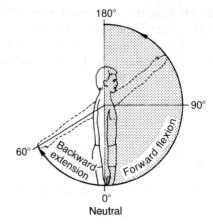

Figure 1.3   Flexion

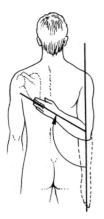

Figure 1.4   Internal rotation

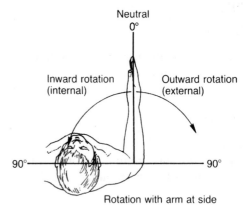

Figure 1.5   External rotation

Pathology in other sites

Examination of the shoulder should always include assessment of the arm, neck and chest, as disorders from these areas may present as a shoulder problem.

COMMON SHOULDER PROBLEMS

Frozen shoulder

This occurs principally in the middle-aged. Generally, there is no apparent precipitating cause, but it may be associated with trauma, cervical spine pathology, diabetes and other metabolic diseases. The characteristic feature of frozen shoulder is a global restriction of movement. Symptoms are probably due to some form of inflammatory process within the capsule of the shoulder joint. The condition tends to be self-limiting, usually lasting no more than 18–36 months. Many patients have heard of the condition, and several will have heard that it is permanently disabling, so it is wise to be reasonably optimistic when describing the diagnosis.

Physiotherapy often aggravates symptoms in the painful phase, but may help when the main problem is stiffness. In particularly troublesome cases intra-articular injection of lidocaine (lignocaine) and an anti-inflammatory agent is often beneficial. Should symptoms persist in a severe form for more than 3–6 months, then referral for a shoulder opinion is indicated. Arthroscopy and manipulation may help in resistant cases.

In this age group, important differential diagnoses are infection and metastatic disease. Impingement symptoms and glenohumeral osteoarthritis can sometimes present with a similar picture to frozen shoulder.

Subacromial impingement (painful arc)

This is a common cause of shoulder symptoms and tends to affect people from age 30 onwards. It is characterized by pain on movement in the shoulder which is worse in particular positions where the greater tuberosity of the humerus impinges against the anterior part of the acromion and the coraco-acromial ligament. It sometimes, but not always, produces a painful arc picture. The symptoms may be bilateral. These symptoms are sometimes associated with rotator cuff tendon tear.

Although the diagnosis can usually be made clinically, plain radiographs of the shoulder may show evidence of beaking of the acromion and bony changes on the humerus. Initial treatment should be by a series of stretching and strengthening exercises. Local anaesthetic and anti-inflammatory injections into the subacromial region through an anterior or posterior approach may

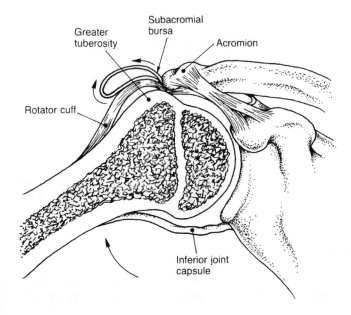

Figure 1.6 The mechanism of impingement of the rotator cuff and subacromial bursa between the humeral head and overlying coracoacromial arch

also be beneficial. Should symptoms persist for more than 3–6 months and be resistant to treatment with physiotherapy and injections, referral is appropriate. Subacromial impingement can be treated surgically with arthroscopic decompression.

Rotator cuff tears

Rotator cuff failure is usually degenerative and begins with the supraspinatus tendon but may extend to include the infraspinatus tendon and subscapularis tendon. It is commonest in the age group 40–60 years. Symptoms are similar to those of subacromial impingement, with pain maximal in certain positions of shoulder movement. Most commonly, this is when the arm is lifted overhead and so it is worth enquiring if the patient can use their arm to reach upwards. Rotator cuff weakness may also be evident on examination and it is particularly important to assess internal and external rotation.

Treatment should begin with a series of stretching and strengthening exercises, followed by injections into the subacromial region if physiotherapy fails to show any benefit. Should symptoms persist, particularly pain, referral is appropriate. Rotator cuff rupture can be successfully treated surgically with acromioplasty and repair of the torn rotator cuff tendon.

Acromioclavicular joint arthritis

This may present in the age group 40 onwards and sometimes follows earlier trauma to the joint. The pain is usually well localized and the joint tender. Treatment with local anaesthetic and steroid injections is frequently successful. Should symptoms persist, surgical excision of the outer end of the clavicle may be an appropriate solution.

Glenohumeral arthritis

Glenohumeral osteoarthritis is less common than arthritis affecting the hip and knee joints. It produces limitations of movement and pain, often occurring at rest and at night. Treatment of early disease with physiotherapy, NSAIDs and steroid injections may help, but if these fail a referral for consideration of total joint replacement should be made.

Bicipital tendonitis

This is an uncommon condition which causes inflammation of the long head of biceps. It is characterized by tenderness in the anterior part of the shoulder and in the bicipital groove of the humerus. Physiotherapy may be beneficial. Occasionally local anaesthetic and steroid injections produce improvement of symptoms. Surgery is very rarely indicated.

Calcifying tendonitis

Calcifying tendonitis is characterized by deposition of calcium deposits within the rotator cuff muscles, usually the supraspinatus. Patients are usually

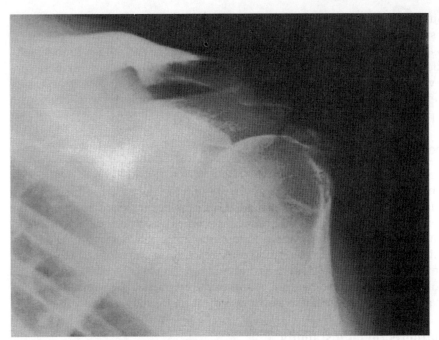

Figure 1.7   X-ray of the shoulder showing calcification of the supraspinatus tendon

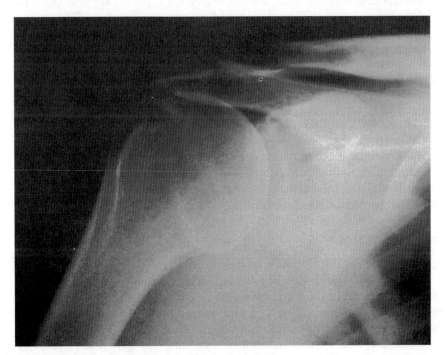

Figure 1.8   Radiograph showing subacromial impingement

younger than those with rotator cuff tears. The symptoms are similar to those of subacromial impingement, with pain and discomfort in certain positions. Treatment should be with physiotherapy to improve the range of movement, followed by local anaesthetic and steroid injections. Treatment with these conservative methods is usually successful, but occasionally surgery is necessary to excise the calcium deposits and perform an acromioplasty. This surgery can be performed arthroscopically.

Recurrent anterior dislocation

These patients are usually in their late teens, twenties or early thirties. Generally there has been trauma to the shoulder in the past, producing either dislocation or subluxation of the joint. If the capsule on the anterior part of the shoulder fails to heal, then the shoulder becomes unstable and liable to recurrent subluxation or dislocation. Symptoms are often intermittent, but the patient is very wary of performing certain activities and often has to give up sport. The best treatment for this condition is surgery with stabilization of the shoulder joint using some form of soft tissue operation. Two episodes of dislocation or subluxation are usually an indication for referral and surgery.

Multidirectional instability

This condition is much less common than traumatic anterior dislocation of the shoulder and it arises from a congenitally lax capsule. There is often no preceding trauma and the shoulder can dislocate in a number of directions. The mainstay of treatment in this condition is physiotherapy and rehabilitation. Referral for advice about appropriate physiotherapy programmes should be offered early. Surgery is only rarely indicated and has a much lower success rate than treatment of anterior dislocations.

Acromioclavicular joint dislocation

This usually occurs in young people following sporting trauma or a fall from a motorbike or a horse. Examination of the joint often shows an obvious deformity. Treatment is with rehabilitation and physiotherapy. If these treatments are unsuccessful, and the dislocation remains painful, then referral to consider surgical reconstruction should be made.

Humeral fractures

Fractures of the proximal humerus in childhood usually involve the neck of the humerus and are invariably treated conservatively. The prognosis is good. In adulthood the commonest fractures are of the neck or of the greater tuberosity, and sometimes internal fixation is required. In the elderly, particularly where bone is osteoporotic, the humerus may fracture into several fragments. Surgical treatment is sometimes necessary. The prognosis should be guarded, as pain and stiffness often occur.

Chapter 2

Elbow

John R. Williams

- A pulled elbow in a child may be treated effectively in primary care without hospital referral.
- Steroid injections for tennis elbow may be repeated for a period of up to 6 months.
- The majority of patients with ulnar nerve entrapment require referral for further investigation.

PRESENTING SYMPTOMS

The elbow joint plays an important role, along with the shoulder and wrist joint, in allowing the arm to place the hand in space. Therefore, consideration of the function and pathology of the elbow must include its interaction with the shoulder, wrist and distal radioulnar joints. Pain and stiffness in the elbow joint can restrict many of the activities of daily living such as eating and personal hygiene.

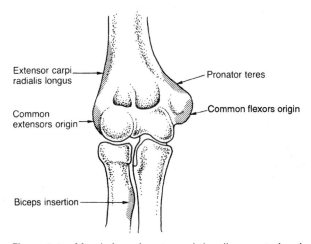

Extensor carpi radialis longus

Pronator teres

Common extensors origin

Common flexors origin

Biceps insertion

Figure 2.1   Muscle insertions around the elbow: anterior view

Assessment of elbow symptoms should distinguish between the three main sites of pathology. These are intra-articular damage and/or loose bodies, peri-articular soft tissue injury and ulnar nerve lesions at the elbow.

Pain

The nature of elbow pain often points to the diagnosis; whether it is constant, including night-time, or if it is related to particular movements or activities. The latter is particularly the case in sports-related injury. The location of the pain can frequently be helpful. Pain from the lateral joint compartment runs up and down the lateral aspect of the arm and forearm. It should be differentiated from shoulder pain or cervical root irritation that may radiate down to the elbow or beyond. Medial pain is more commonly associated with medial epicondylitis (golfer's elbow), ulnar nerve entrapment or arthritis.

PHYSICAL EXAMINATION

When examining the elbow it is important to also consider the neck, shoulder, wrist and distal radioulnar joints.

Inspect

Muscle wasting, gross deformity, soft tissue swelling and effusions can all be visible on inspection. Deformity is best displayed with the elbow in the

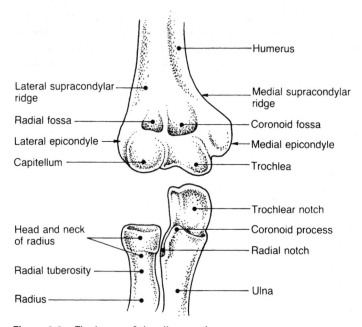

Figure 2.2   The bones of the elbow region

extended position, remembering that the normal carrying angle is 10–15 degrees of valgus. Deformities here are commonly caused by intra-articular pathology or growth disturbance following a childhood fracture.

Palpate

Palpation of the elbow region should include four aspects. Laterally, one can examine the supracondylar ridge and lateral epicondyle, the lateral joint margins and radial head. The radial head can be fully examined around its edge by rotation of the forearm. Medially, the medial epicondyle is felt. Behind it the ulnar nerve can be rolled underneath the examiner's finger. The origin of the flexor–pronator group of muscles can be palpated. Posteriorly, examination should include the olecranon, its bursa and the triceps tendon. Anteriorly, the most important structure is the biceps tendon and its insertions.

Move

Movements of the elbow joint occur around two axes. The first is flexion and extension, which range from 0 to 140 degrees. The second is rotation around the forearm axis. The normal range of rotation is 75 degrees of pronation and 85 degrees of supination (with the shoulder fixed to prevent abduction or adduction). Intra-articular disorders often cause reduction in passive extension or rotation. If there is a reduction in the range of movement, assess whether the end point is firm or soft.

The stability of the medial and lateral collateral ligaments can be tested. The medial ligament is tested by exerting a valgus force on the forearm after the elbow has been flexed to 15 degrees to relax the anterior capsule. Similarly, the lateral ligament is tested by a varus stress in the same position of flexion.

Locking

This is relatively uncommon in primary care; however, it has different causes in different age groups. The locking is usually loss of extension and occurs intermittently. In young adults it is usually caused by a single loose body following intra-articular trauma or occasionally osteochondritis dissecans. In older patients it is due to osteoarthritis or occasionally synovial chondromatosis.

Table 2.1   Normal range of movement: elbow

Flexion	0–150 degrees
Pronation	0–75 degrees
Supination	0–85 degrees

COMMON ELBOW PROBLEMS

Children

The majority of conditions around the child's elbow follow trauma. A number of congenital disorders affect the elbow, but these are rare. Both cerebral palsy and haemophilia may occasionally affect the elbow.

Pulled elbow

One traumatic elbow condition which may occasionally present to general practitioners is the 'pulled elbow' or 'nursemaid's elbow'. This is usually caused by swinging the child around by the extended arms (or other similar action causing axial forces along the extended arm) and results in the radial head slipping under the edge of the annular ligament. The child is commonly between 6 months and 3 years old and accompanied by the distraught adult involved. It rarely has any sinister connotations with non-accidental injury. The elbow is painful and the child will resist movement from the pronated and flexed position. It can be treated by quickly supinating the forearm with

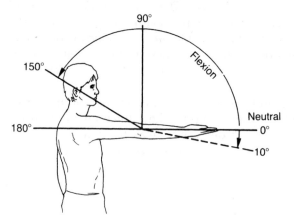

Figure 2.3   Flexion and extension

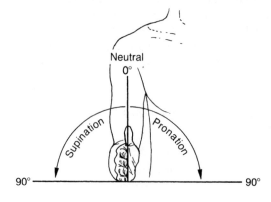

Figure 2.4   Pronation and supination

axial and valgus strain while still in the flexed position. This screws the radial head back through the annular ligament into its normal position. The relocation is often accompanied by a click or pop and immediate relief of pain in the child and anguish in the adult. Immobilization is not required afterwards.

ADULTS

Overuse conditions

Overuse conditions are common in primary care. They may be acute or chronic, occurring usually in patients who are between 30 and 55 years old.

Tennis elbow

This condition is sometimes known as lateral epicondylitis. Although tennis elbow may be seen in tennis players, this is relatively rare. It is common in other sports players and occupations that involve repetitive forearm activities such as using a keyboard. The pain is localized to the lateral side of the elbow around the origin of extensor group of muscles. Most cases are unilateral, but 10–20% of cases are bilateral. Those cases that are non-occupational and are caused by one particular and isolated activity, such as clipping the hedge, will usually resolve without any treatment other than reassurance and analgesia.

Treatment within the first few months is advisable, as delays worsen the prognosis. The mainstays of this treatment are rest, pain relief, splintage and injection of the affected area. Rest involves modifying the activity thought to be causing the problem. This may be aided by equipment adjustment, such as changing the handle size of the racket, altering the training regime or correction of position during work. For pain relief NSAIDs are generally effective. Various arm braces have been used; however, the smaller ones rarely stay in the correct position and the more substantial and effective ones are often unacceptable to the patient. Physiotherapy is not particularly beneficial. If these methods fail a simple injection of local anaesthetic and steroid is indicated. Superficial injection should be avoided, as not only is it ineffective but also it may cause skin atrophy. Injections may be carried out at 6-weekly to 2-monthly intervals. However, if this frequency of injection is required for more than 6 months then other treatments should be sought. Regular injections every 4–6 months, provided that they are placed deeply, are safe. If all these methods fail referral for consideration of surgery should be offered. Surgery consists of release of the extensor origin. Following surgery the arm should not be immobilized for more than 1 week. Then gentle strengthening exercises can begin with a planned return to sport or activity at a mild level at 6 weeks.

Golfer's elbow

This is medial epicondylitis occurring in the common flexor origin, and is analogous to tennis elbow occurring on the medial side. Treatment is similar, with the proviso that injections must avoid the ulnar nerve lying behind the medial epicondyle. Golfer's elbow may be confused with nerve symptoms from entrapment at the neck, elbow or wrist.

Rheumatoid arthritis

The elbow is frequently affected in rheumatoid arthritis. The rheumatoid elbow should never be viewed in isolation without reference to the shoulder, wrist and hand.

As well as the joint being affected by the destructive arthritis, there may also be rheumatoid nodules and involvement of the olecranon bursa. Proliferation of the synovium can compromise the function of the nerves at the elbow. Up to half of patients with rheumatoid arthritis develop elbow problems, the majority of which follow a slow, chronic path.

Rest, splintage and physiotherapy are frequently helpful. The use of analgesics, non-steroidal anti-inflammatories, corticosteroid injections and disease-modifying drugs may be required. Patients will usually be managed jointly with a rheumatologist, and sometimes an orthopaedic surgeon.

Osteoarthritis

Elbow osteoarthritis is far less common than that of the hip or knee. The majority are secondary to trauma. Post-traumatic arthritis of the elbow is increasing in incidence particularly in patients aged between 40 and 50 years.

Patients have pain in the joint, often on the lateral side, specifically with activity but also at night. There is tenderness around the radial head and along the edge of the ulnar–humeral articulation. There is often a subtle decrease in range of movement, particularly passive terminal extension. Intermittent locking of the joint with pain suggests the development of intra-articular loose bodies. Radiographs confirm the diagnosis.

Initial treatment is symptomatic with analgesics and exercises, followed by joint injection if required. Surgical intervention using arthroscopic techniques allows visualization of the articular surfaces, washout, removal of small loose bodies and limited debridement. Good results are reported after open debridement. Total joint replacement is an option in these patients; however, in patients with high demands on their elbows the success rates are less encouraging than in the rheumatoid patient.

Post-traumatic contracture

This problem generally follows trauma. In the acute situation it should be tackled immediately with physiotherapy and splintage. If these fail and the contracture causes a functional problem then anterior capsulotomy, either arthroscopically or open, may be required.

Olecranon bursitis

This may be traumatic, infective or inflammatory. It is commonly seen in primary care and on most occasions does not require treatment. Traumatic bursitis may follow a single injury or be due to repeated insult: the so-called student's or miner's elbow. It can be difficult to differentiate between septic and inflammatory bursitis. A history of fever, marked tenderness and overlying cellulitis favour an infective cause. A full blood count and aspiration will help in the diagnosis when doubt exists. Radiographs are only helpful in diagnosing an olecranon spur. Septic bursae can be aspirated, followed by rest, elevation and antibiotics. Occasionally surgical drainage may be needed.

Non-septic bursae can usually be treated symptomatically and the patient advised to avoid rubbing the elbow. Many practitioners achieve satisfactory results in small and moderate bursae by aspiration and injection of steroids, followed by compression. If the bursa becomes a chronic problem, excision can be undertaken. This is often an extensive procedure.

Ulnar nerve entrapment

The most common site of ulnar nerve entrapment is in the cubital tunnel behind the medial epicondyle. This presents as pain down the medial side of the forearm extending into the ulnar digits. Pain may also extend upwards on the medial side of the arm. The pain is a dull, gnawing ache with associated paraesthesiae. Sensory changes can be detected in the ulnar digits with reduced two-point discrimination and later motor weakness, often initially seen in the first dorsal interosseous muscle. Referral to a specialist is appropriate. The majority of patients require surgery following electrophysiological confirmation of the site of the lesion.

Chapter 3

Hand and wrist

Peter Burge

- Seventy per cent of trigger fingers are asymptomatic 1 year after a single injection of steroid.
- The majority of ganglions of the hand and wrist can be managed in primary care.
- Painful hand infections require prompt referral and surgical drainage.
- Dupuytren's disease without contracture is not an indication for referral.

PRESENTING SYMPTOMS

The presentation of hand and wrist problems is very variable. It may include symptoms of pain and restriction of movement, but may also involve neurological symptoms or more specific problems such as those encountered in trigger finger. The hand is also particularly prone to trauma and to infections. It is important to be aware of acute pain and swelling as possible markers of a hand infection which requires urgent treatment.

PHYSICAL EXAMINATION

Inspect

Inspection of the hand may reveal swelling or deformity. Ganglia are the most common cause of swelling in the hand and wrist, usually occurring on the posterior surface of the wrist. Deformities of the hand may be due to local problems such as Dupuytren's contracture. However, they may also be due to arthritis.

Palpation

Feeling the hand and wrist may pinpoint the location of pain and tenderness. It may also reveal swellings of underlying tissues as in trigger finger. Examination should also include a neurological examination.

Move

Examination of passive and active movement of the wrist and digits is important to determine if any weakness or fixed deformity is present. Formal assessment of grip and pinch grip strength may sometimes be of value.

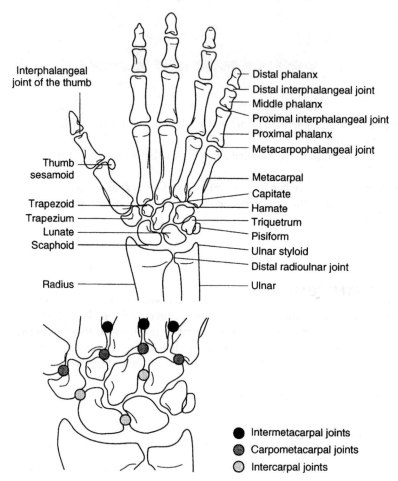

Interphalangeal
joint of the thumb

Distal phalanx
Distal interphalangeal joint
Middle phalanx
Proximal interphalangeal joint
Proximal phalanx
Metacarpophalangeal joint

Thumb
sesamoid

Metacarpal

Capitate
Trapezoid — Hamate
Trapezium — Triquetrum
Lunate — Pisiform
Scaphoid — Ulnar styloid
Distal radioulnar joint

Radius — Ulnar

● Intermetacarpal joints
◓ Carpometacarpal joints
◯ Intercarpal joints

Figure 3.1   The bones and joints of the wrist and hand

Table 3.1   Normal range of movement: wrist

Extension	0–70 degrees
Flexion	0–80 degrees
Radial deviation	0–20 degrees
Ulnar deviation	0–30 degrees

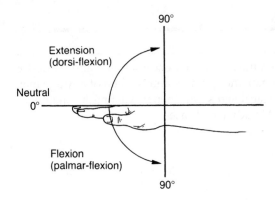

Figure 3.2   Flexion and extension of the wrist

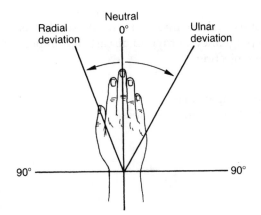

Figure 3.3   Radial and ulnar deviation of the wrist

Table 3.2   Normal range of movement: fingers

Flexion	
DIP joint	0–90 degrees
PIP joint	0–100 degrees
MCP joint	0–90 degrees

Table 3.3   Normal range of movement: thumb

Flexion	
IP joint	0–80 degrees
MCP joint	0–50 degrees
CMC joint	0–15 degrees
Abduction	0–70 degrees

COMMON HAND PROBLEMS

Carpal tunnel syndrome

The diagnosis is usually clear from the history of nocturnal pain and paraesthesiae affecting a middle-aged woman, though men and women of any age may be affected. There may be no physical signs, but thenar wasting, weakness or sensory impairment can be found in advanced cases.

Treatments in primary care include:

- *Rest*: avoid provoking activities if possible.
- *Night splintage*: prevents wrist flexion during sleep (flexion increases pressure in the carpal tunnel). Use a Futuro or similar splint.
- *Diuretics*: there is no evidence to support the use of diuretics.
- *Steroid injection*: 80% of patients respond, but 80% have a recurrence within 2 years.

Recurrence is less likely if the history is short. Injection is most useful when resolution can be expected, as with pregnancy, or thyroid disease. It is important to avoid the median nerve when injecting.

Indications for referral are:

- thenar wasting or constant sensory impairment
- moderate symptoms without objective neurological loss

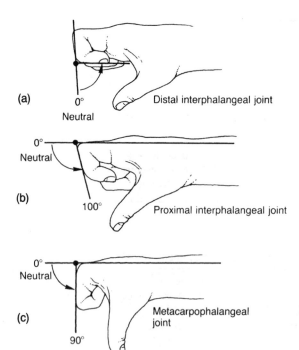

Figure 3.4   Finger flexion: (a) distal interphalangeal joint; (b) proximal interphalangeal joint; (c) metacarpophalangeal joint

- failure of a 3-month trial of conservative treatment
- severe symptoms without neurological loss.

Trigger finger/thumb

Trigger finger is characterized by locking or catching of a finger during active flexion. It may be associated with rheumatoid arthritis or diabetes. Treatment

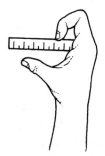

Fingertip to
distal palmar crease

(a)

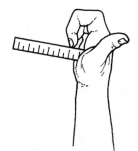

Fingertip to
proximal palmar crease

(b)

Figure 3.5   (a), (b)
Composite motion of flexion

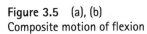

Zero starting position

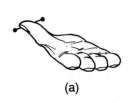

(a)

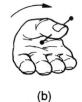

(b)

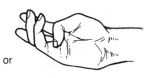

Flexion to tip of
little finger

or

Flexion to base of
little finger

(c)

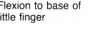

Figure 3.6   Thumb
movements: (a) Extension,
(b) Opposition, (c) Flexion

Table 3.4   Common causes of wrist and hand pain in different age groups

| Age group | Cause | | |
	Intra-articular	Periarticular	Referred
Childhood (2–10 years)	Infection	Fracture Osteomyelitis	
Adolescence (10–18 years)	Infection	Trauma Osteomyelitis Tumours Ganglion Idiopathic wrist pain	
Early adulthood (18–30 years)	Inflammatory arthritis Infection	Peripheral nerve entrapment Tendonitis Ganglion	Cervical
Adulthood (30–50 years)	Inflammatory arthritis Infection Osteoarthritis	Peripheral nerve entrapment Tendonitis	Cervical Chest Cardiac
Old age (>50 years)	Inflammatory arthritis Osteoarthritis	Peripheral nerve entrapment Tendonitis	Cervical Chest Cardiac

in primary care should include night splintage of the interphalangeal joints in extension (a tongue depressor and tape will suffice) and steroid injection of the flexor tendon sheath. About 70% of trigger digits remain asymptomatic 1 year after a single injection. Indications for referral are persistent or recurrent triggering after one injection or doubt about the diagnosis.

De Quervain's syndrome

This causes pain and swelling over the styloid process of the radius, usually after strenuous activity, and is due to thickening of the abductor pollicis longus tendon sheath. Pain is aggravated by active extension of the thumb. Finkelstein's test is diagnostic. The thumb is flexed into the palm and grasped by the fingers; the examiner then moves the wrist into ulnar deviation causing pain along the tendon sheath. It should be compared to the normal side.

Treatments in primary care include:

- *Rest*: avoid provoking activities if possible.
- *Splintage*: the splint should include the thumb as a simple wrist splint is not effective.
- *NSAIDs*.
- *Steroid injection*: this is highly effective. Avoid placing steroid in the subcutaneous tissues, where it may cause atrophy.

Ganglion

1. Dorsal wrist ganglion, over the scapholunate ligament.
2. Palmar wrist ganglion, adjacent to the radial artery.
3. Palmar digital ganglion, from the flexor tendon sheath at the base of the finger.

Ganglia are common and harmless. About 40% resolve spontaneously over 10 years. Teenagers and young adults are most often affected. Patients seek advice because of pain, an unsightly swelling or concern over the diagnosis. Pain and swelling often fluctuate.

Many patients with ganglia require only explanation and reassurance that the lesion is harmless and that it may resolve spontaneously. Surgical scars at the wrist may be as unattractive as the original problem and excision does not always relieve pain. The recurrence rate after surgery is about 5–10% for dorsal wrist ganglia, 45% for ganglia adjacent to the radial artery and almost nil for palmar digital ganglia.

Treatment in primary care should involve explanation and reassurance. Aspiration of wrist ganglia is also possible. About 20% disappear for at least 12 months after aspiration with a wide bore needle under local anaesthesia. After simple puncture of palmar digital ganglia with a 21-gauge needle, the recurrence rate is under 25%.

Indications for referral are a large or persistently painful dorsal wrist ganglion. Indications for excision of palmar wrist ganglia are limited, as the recurrence rate is high. Painful palmar digital ganglia may persist or recur after needle puncture and require excision.

Wrist pain

There are many causes of wrist pain, some of which need surgical management. In most cases, pain is self-limiting and responds to simple measures such as support bandaging, rest, analgesics and physiotherapy. Referral is appropriate only if these measures have failed, or if radiographs are abnormal. Patients who have normal movement, strong grip and normal plain radiographs seldom have surgically treatable pathology.

Treatment in primary care should include analgesia, particularly NSAIDs, support bandaging and rest. Plain radiographs are useful in excluding underlying pathology. Indications for referral are persistent pain and abnormal plain radiographs.

Osteoarthritis of basal thumb joint

This condition affects about 15% of the older female population. It is often asymptomatic. Management in primary care involves explanation and reassurance, analgesia and splintage. Steroid injection often helps: distract the joint by traction and walk the needle off the base of the metacarpal into the joint. The indication for referral is persistent pain, not responding to these measures.

Osteoarthritis of distal interphalangeal joint (Heberden's nodes)

Persistent pain is uncommon. Women are much more commonly affected than men. The nodes are often familial. Pain tends to subside with time, leaving the joints swollen and a little stiff, but good function is usually preserved. It is important to emphasize this as many patients fear they will lose good use of their hands. Management in primary care involves advice and analgesia. Persistent pain is an indication for referral. Fusion is the only satisfactory surgical option.

Dupuytren's disease

This disease is common and often hereditary. Alcohol, smoking, diabetes and anticonvulsant medication are risk factors. Treatment in primary care involves explanation and reassurance. Indications for referral are an inability to place the hand flat on the table and any contracture of the proximal interphalangeal joint. If there is no contracture, referral is unlikely to be of value.

Hand infections

Early soft tissue infections, before pus has formed, usually respond to antibiotics; the most common infecting organism is *Staphylococcus aureus*. Pain preventing sleep indicates pus and is an indication for surgical drainage in hospital. Fluctuation appears late in the hand and is not useful in early diagnosis. The most important issue is to consider the possibility of deep infection. Failure to respond to antibiotics over 24–48 hours, as well as pain preventing sleep, are indications to refer to hospital urgently. Beware of the apparent cellulitis which is in fact a deeper abscess.

Any penetrating wound over a tendon sheath or joint should be regarded with suspicion. Flexor tendon sheath infection and septic arthritis develop over a few hours and can ruin the tendon or joint. These infections should be treated by urgent surgical drainage – antibiotics are only an adjunct to surgery. Animal bites and human tooth wounds are particularly liable to infection and frequently penetrate joints.

COMMON HAND INJURIES

Fractures

Any hand injury followed by swelling or bruising may be a fracture. The only safe rule is to organize an X-ray, as opportunities for treatment may be lost by delay. Most fractures need no treatment other than taping to an adjacent finger, but serious injuries cannot be distinguished from trivial injuries without X-rays.

Mallet finger

This is a loss of active extension of the distal interphalangeal joint due to traumatic rupture of the extensor tendon, usually after a stubbing type of injury.

The treatment is immediate splintage in extension continued for 6–8 weeks. Apply a temporary splint and refer the patient.

Lacerations

Lacerations often conceal injuries to nerves or tendons that can be missed unless the appropriate physical signs are elicited. All structures passing near the laceration should be assumed to be divided until their integrity has been demonstrated by examination. If integrity cannot be demonstrated (small child, uncooperative adult), the wound should be explored in hospital.

Subungual haematoma

This problem is usually due to a crush injury which fractures the tuft of the terminal phalanx. Evacuation of the haematoma by piercing the nail with a hot wire relieves pain, but is usually unnecessary.

Chapter 4

Cervical spine
Jeremy C. T. Fairbank

- Neck instability is an important symptom usually reflecting serious pathology.
- Most patients with cervical spondylosis respond to conservative treatment.
- A patient with a history of trauma and neck symptoms who has already had a cervical spine X-ray may require a further X-ray examination.
- Sixty per cent of whiplash injuries respond within 3 months – litigation has an adverse effect on outcome.

PRESENTING SYMPTOMS

Neck problems may present with pain, stiffness, neurological deficit and occasionally clicking, snapping or sensations of instability.

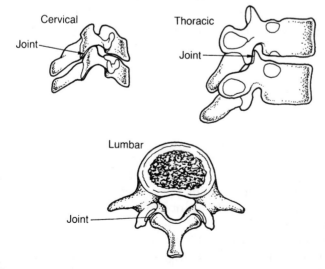

Figure 4.1   Regional differences between vertebrae

Pain

Pain is commonly intermittent and related to activity. Rest pain or night pain should be taken seriously and may be due to a tumour or infection. It is an indication for taking a plain radiograph if it continues for more than 6 weeks.

Pain may be experienced in the midline, and may radiate distally, but usually to no more than two segments. Pain may radiate into the shoulders and arms by two mechanisms. One is the familiar root pain where symptoms are experienced in a typical dermatomal distribution. The other is referred pain, which is much less easy to define although extremely commonly experienced. This is frequently felt in the shoulder or upper arm and tends to radiate further down the arm the worse the pain is. This pain is referred in a 'sclerodermal' fashion in the distribution of the innervation of muscle. This type of pain arises in all parts of the spine but is particularly obvious in pain from the neck and low back. Referred pain may be accompanied by local tenderness at the source of radiating pain as well as in the distribution of that pain. These 'trigger points' have also been called 'fibrositis' or 'tender points' and can be helped on occasion by injections of local anaesthetic or acupuncture.

Pain may develop acutely or chronically. Patients frequently have difficulty in describing pain, but it may be experienced in the distributions described above. It is worth examining the cervical spine for tenderness to see whether or not you can reproduce pain from a specific level. You may also find tender points distributed over the back, scapulae, shoulders or in the arms. Quite how important these tender points are remains controversial. Pain from the neck is sometimes difficult to distinguish clinically from pain arising from the shoulder or arm. Often movement of the shoulder, elbow or wrist will reproduce the pain and so suggest a source away from the cervical spine for the problem.

Stiffness

This frequently, but not always, accompanies pain. It is not usually helpful in establishing the diagnosis, but may relate to the patient's perception of disability.

Neurological symptoms and signs

Pain, paraesthesia, weakness and loss of function may present in a dermatomal distribution. This often, although not always, reflects significant neurological damage, and must always be taken seriously. Cervical myelopathy may present insidiously and is not always easy to diagnose. The patient may describe difficulties with walking and unsteadiness when standing. In the arms, pain, weakness and loss of dexterity may be experienced. The classic dermatomes are illustrated in Figure 4.2. The distribution of motor signs relating to nerve roots is shown in Figure 4.3.

Patients with cervical myelopathy may exhibit Lhermitte's sign. This is a sensation of 'electric shocks' on flexion or extension of the neck. These electric

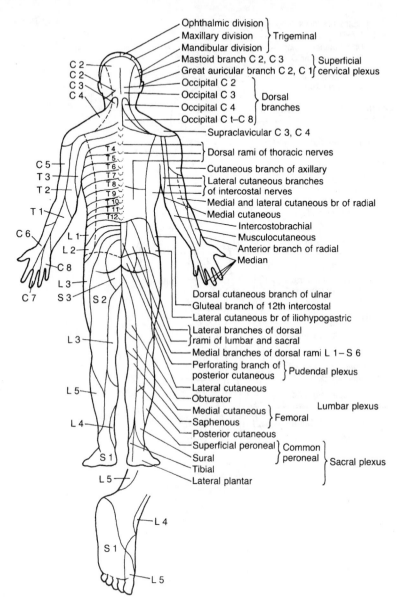

Figure 4.2   Dermatomes (cutaneous distribution of spinal segments and peripheral nerves): posterior aspect

shocks or paraesthesiae may be experienced in all four limbs as well as over the top of the head. There may be disturbance of the normal deep tendon relaxes and occasionally a positive Hoffman's sign (flicking of the palmar surface of the middle finger causing flexion of the thumb and index finger). Bladder and bowel dysfunction should be enquired after, but are not always experienced in patients with chronic myelopathy.

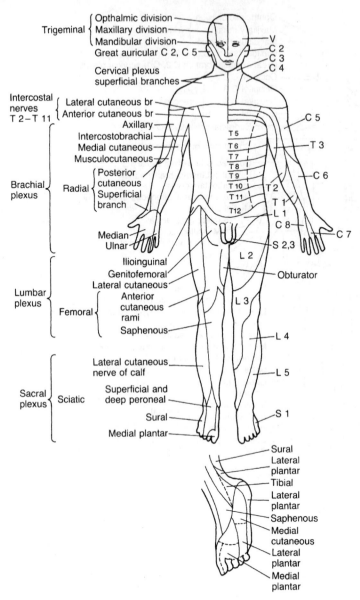

Figure 4.3 Dermatomes (cutaneous distribution of spinal segments and peripheral nerves): anterior aspect

Instability

This occurs when the neck is rendered unstable by trauma, tumours or destructive arthropathies (rheumatoid arthritis, osteoarthritis, ankylosing spondylitis, etc.). This symptom must always be taken seriously.

Instability means a sensation that the patient does not normally experience. Patients feel that their head is no longer firmly fixed to the rest of the body,

Table 4.1   Normal range of movement: neck

Flexion	0–45 degrees
Extension	0–45 degrees
Lateral flexion	0–45 degrees
Rotation	0–60 degrees

or that any movements engender a sensation of panic. At its extreme, patients may support their head with their hands. They may find their symptoms difficult to describe, as they are something new and unfamiliar. On occasion neck pain may be associated with sensations of dizziness.

PHYSICAL EXAMINATION

Look for the position and range of movement of the cervical spine, as well as torticollis or muscle wasting.

Neurological examination

Perform a neurological examination of the upper limbs, including tests of sensation, power and reflexes. If you suspect cervical spine pathology then also observe the gait and examine the legs neurologically.

A rapid screen of the upper limbs involves resisted abduction of the shoulders, flexion and extension of the elbow, dorsiflexion of the wrist, abduction of the fingers and abduction of the thumbs.

MANAGEMENT

If there is a clear-cut history of trauma, then obtain a radiograph to exclude bony pathology and refer for physiotherapy assessment after a negative X-ray. You should not be afraid of requesting a further radiograph even if a patient has already had one, as late subluxation from soft tissue injuries to the neck is well recognized and sometimes fractures are missed at the initial examination. In case of doubt refer to an orthopaedic surgeon.

If there is no history of trauma and the pain is intermittent, NSAIDs followed by a trial of a soft collar or physiotherapy are the initial management. Soft collars are sometimes best worn at night and it is worth the patient experimenting with this. As far as possible one should avoid prolonged immobilization in the collar.

If the pain is continuous with night pain, request a radiograph and consider tumour and infection. This may be an indication for referral to a specialist.

If there are definite signs or clear neurological symptoms, obtain radiograph and refer urgently to an orthopaedic surgeon or a neurosurgeon. Similarly, sensations of instability should be taken seriously and are probably an indication for urgent referral to an orthopaedic surgeon.

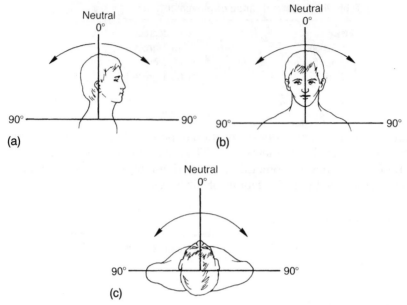

Figure 4.4   (a) Flexion; (b) lateral flexion; (c) rotation

COMMON CERVICAL PROBLEMS

Torticollis

This is due to contraction of one sternomastoid muscle, giving a characteristic 'wry neck'. It is common in infants, and normally responds to stretching by a parent under health visitor or physiotherapist supervision. In older children and adults it may occur spontaneously or after a minor injury (acute rotatory subluxation). There is a spectrum of complaints, from the minor, which can be managed by reassurance and rest, to more severe symptoms which should probably be referred to a specialist. A very severe torticollis responds to inpatient traction and physiotherapy and is, therefore, an indication for emergency referral. Some patients with minor stiffness will respond to manipulative treatment from a physiotherapist or a qualified alternative practitioner.

Cervical spondylosis

This is a generic term which covers a wide range of common disorders of the cervical spine. The pathology is degenerative changes in the cervical intervertebral discs and their adjacent synovial joints (the joints of Luschka). These joints are exclusively present in the neck and are one of the reasons why rheumatoid arthritis produces serious problems in the cervical spine, but less commonly elsewhere in the spine. The facet or apophyseal joints are also synovial and may be involved in rheumatoid arthritis.

Table 4.2 Primary management of cervical spondylosis associated with arm pain

Advice and education	Reassurance
	Rest
	Occupation
	Psychotherapy
Physiotherapy	Heat/cold
Chiropractic	Exercises
Osteopathy	Acupuncture
	TENS
	Traction
Drugs	Analgesics
	NSAIDs
	Injections

Cervical spondylosis is frequently asymptomatic and may be detected by minor changes on plain radiographs. Indeed, there is very little correlation between the severity of radiological changes and the severity of the patient's symptoms, so in most cases a radiograph is unnecessary. However, on occasion a radiograph may be of therapeutic value to explain the process to patients and for reassurance.

In some patients the persistence and severity of pain may require referral, assuming simple measures such as a collar, NSAIDs or physiotherapy have been ineffective. In more severe cases the disease process may cause nerve root pain by nerve root irritation or compression. In the worst circumstances, particularly if the patient has the misfortune to be born with a narrow cervical canal, it may lead to cervical myelopathy, as described above. However, most patients with cervical spondylosis respond to conservative measures and do not require specialist referral. There is a small minority of patients with chronic cervical pain who respond to cervical fusion. This operation also allows nerve root decompression. Depending on local circumstances, this may be performed by neurosurgeons or orthopaedic surgeons. Cervical spondylosis may be a cause of headaches but this symptom should be handled within the normal differential diagnosis for headaches and is outside the scope of this book.

Cervical fractures

While most of these are recognized acutely and are managed by the emergency services, diagnosis of serious injury may be delayed because:

1. the original injury was missed
2. the severity only becomes apparent after the general practitioner has requested a radiograph, usually because of persisting or increasing pain

3. a late deformity has developed

4. there is a progressive neurological deficit.

These patients require immediate referral for specialist management, usually by an orthopaedic surgeon.

'Whiplash' injuries

Neck pain following even minor road traffic accidents is common. Prolonged symptoms may occur, especially in the aggrieved party. Fractures can usually be identified on radiographs taken in the accident and emergency department, but soft tissue injures and consequent instability may be missed. If in doubt in the face of persisting symptoms, repeat films are helpful (say a week or two following the original injury). The vast majority of low speed rear-end collisions do not have identifiable injuries, even with sophisticated scanners.

Unfortunately, a variety of trials of interventions (collars, physiotherapy, chiropractic, manipulation, analgesics, etc.) have not demonstrated any real advantage over natural history. Most patients see significant symptom reduction by 4 weeks, and many will go on for 3–6 months. Those still with symptoms at this stage almost invariably are involved in litigation. Several studies have shown that those with symptoms at 1 year will persist indefinitely. There is some evidence that symptoms are stronger and more prolonged in a soft tissue injured population than those with identified fractures. Risk factors are pre-existing cervical spondylosis and a previous history of neck pain (which is why experts are so anxious to review the whole GP record of a patient).

It is important to document an indication of the energy of the accident (by damage to vehicle), and the timing and nature of symptom onset. Low back pain may also occur. Examination of neck tenderness, movement and any neurological signs should be documented. This is helpful not only medically but also for the legal process that frequently follows.

Management should be by explanation (muscle and ligament strain), analgesics and encouraging early mobilization. Soft collars are best avoided. Community physiotherapists should be supporting the same line. *The Whiplash Book* (Burton K, McClune T, Waddell G 2002 *The Whiplash Book: How You Can Deal With a Whiplash Injury*, Stationery Office Books, London), is helpful to give, sell or rent to patients. So far no trial of this intervention has been published, but in my view the advice is sound.

Cervical disc prolapse

This is less common than a lumbar disc prolapse. It usually affects the central segments of the cervical spine. Root pain is usually preceded by a variable period of neck pain. Neurological signs in the distribution of the affected nerve root may be present. In most cases these settle down with analgesia and

Table 4.3   Factors associated with persistent and severe whiplash injuries

Severe whiplash injury
High-speed injury
Intense and rapid onset of pain
Severe restriction of movement at presentation
Abnormal neurology
Bony injuries

Persistent whiplash injury
High-speed injury
Intense and rapid onset of pain
Severe restriction of movement at presentation
Abnormal neurology
Bony injuries
Increasing age
Upper limb paraesthesiae
Cervical spondylosis

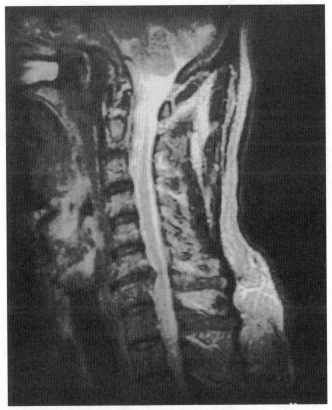

Figure 4.5   MRI showing a prolapsed cervical disc

the symptoms resolve. Steroids may be of value with persistent pain, but this is controversial. If there is a progressive neurological deficit, seek a specialist opinion.

Cervical myelopathy

This is insidious in onset with unsteadiness of gait, upper limb clumsiness and sometimes pain. It is managed by neurosurgeons or specialist orthopaedic spine surgeons.

Chapter **5**

Lumbar spine
James Wilson-MacDonald

- Mechanical low back pain is best treated by early mobilization and physiotherapy.
- Back pain which is unremitting or associated with urinary and bowel symptoms or with weakness requires urgent referral.
- Twenty per cent of asymptomatic individuals will have evidence of disc prolapse on an MRI scan.
- Characteristic features of spinal stenosis in the elderly include leg pain induced by walking, relieved by sitting and associated with numbness and paraesthesiae.

PRESENTING SYMPTOMS

It is important to differentiate between the conditions requiring referral and those where conservative measures such as physiotherapy should be used initially.

Pain and neurological symptoms

Symptoms which may require urgent referral include night pain of a constant nature, constant unremitting pain, urinary or bowel symptoms, or symptoms of weakness. Constant unremitting pain is suggestive of either malignancy or infection and these patients are best seen as early as possible. Referral either immediately or within a few days is indicated, depending on the severity of the symptoms. Patients who present with weakness in the limbs or with urological or bowel symptoms may have compression either of the nerve root or of the spinal cord, so urgent referral is indicated.

Chronic pain

The more chronic symptoms which most patients describe, such as low back pain, and mild or intermittent neurological symptoms in the legs, do not

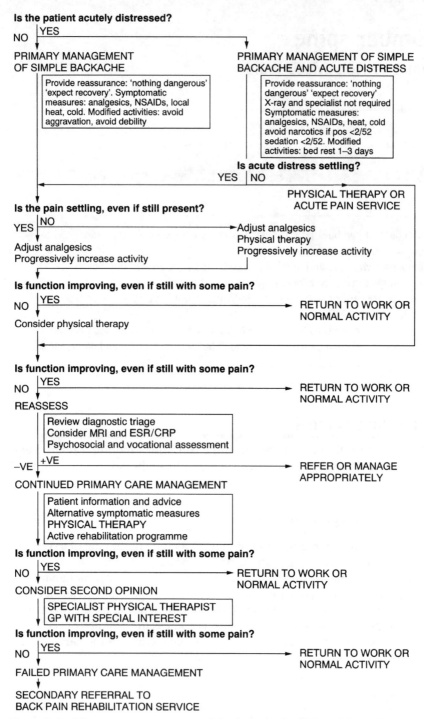

Figure 5.1   Primary care management of simple backache. (Adapted from Clinical Standards Advisory Group 1994 *Back Pain*, HMSO, London)

Initial consultation

Diagnostic triage	• Simple backache	
	• Nerve root pain	} urgent
	• Serious spinal pathology	} referral

Early management strategy:

Aims: symptomatic relief of pain; prevent disability

Prescribe simple analgesia, NSAIDs
- avoid narcotics if possible and never more than 2 weeks

Arrange physical therapy if symptoms last more than a few days
- manipulation
- active exercise and physical activity – modifies pain mechanisms, speeds recovery

Advise rest only if essential: 1–3 days
- prolonged bed rest is harmful

Encourage early activity
- activity is beneficial
- reduces pain
- physical fitness beneficial

Practise psychosocial management; this is fundamental
- promote positive attitudes to activity and work
- distress and depression

Advise absence from work only if unavoidable; early return to work
- prolonged sickness absence makes return to work increasingly difficult

Biopsychosocial assessment at 6 weeks

Review diagnostic triage
ESR/CRP and MRI scan lumbosacral spine if specifically indicated
Psychosocial and vocational assessment

Active rehabilitation programme

Incremental aerobic exercise and fitness programme of physical reconditioning
Behavioural medicine principles
Close liaison with the workplace

Secondary referral

Second opinion
Rehabilitation
Vocational assessment and guidance
Surgery
Pain management

Final outcome measure: maintain productive activity; reduce work loss

Figure 5.2   An overview of management guidelines for acute back pain. (Adapted from Clinical Standards Advisory Group 1994 *Back Pain*, HMSO, London)

require such urgent referral. Indeed most of these patients benefit from a period of delay in that many of them resolve spontaneously. Conservative treatment especially in the form of physiotherapy may make referral unnecessary. Every patient referred to hospital with mechanical low back pain should have had physiotherapy prior to referral to hospital.

PHYSICAL EXAMINATION

Inspect

Observation of the way the patient moves about and dresses and undresses is helpful in confirming the severity of symptoms. Observation of the back may reveal muscle spasm or a deformity of the spine. Often the deformity is due to a so-called sciatic scoliosis; when the patient lies down, the deformity resolves. Fixed deformities are suggestive of true scoliosis or severe degenerative changes. There may be muscle wasting in the lower limbs, although this is unusual except in chronic conditions.

Palpate

Palpation will reveal the area of tenderness in the spine, and can help to some extent with identifying the level of the lesion.

Move

The sciatic and femoral stretch tests may be positive if there is nerve root compression. The femoral stretch test is performed with the patient prone and the knee flexed. A positive test is shown by pain down the front of the thigh, when the hip is extended. The sciatic stretch test is performed with the patient supine. The hip and knee are flexed to 90 degrees, and the knee is then gently straightened. A positive response will elicit pain down the back of the leg. The hip may need to be extended to allow full knee extension, and the angle of hip flexion will be the straight leg raise angle.

Neurology

Reflex changes are also useful in isolating the level of nerve root compression, although there may be variation in the nerve root supply of any single reflex, and these are not necessarily reliable. Lesions such as disc prolapses may also affect more than one nerve root.

Signs of neurological impairment

If the patient has bowel or urinary symptoms, or there is significant nerve root pain or spinal cord compression is suspected, then rectal examination and examination of perineal sensation is essential. Reduced anal tone or altered sensation in the perineum may be suggestive of a central cord lesion in the lower lumbar spine. Upper motor neurone signs in the lower limbs suggest a lesion compressing the spinal cord more proximally. These signs include upgoing plantars, clonus, and difficulty with balance and weakness in the lower limbs due to impaired proprioception.

Table 5.1   Normal range of movement: thoracolumbar spine

Flexion	0–80 degrees
Extension	0–20 degrees
Lateral bend	0–35 degrees
Rotation	0–45 degrees

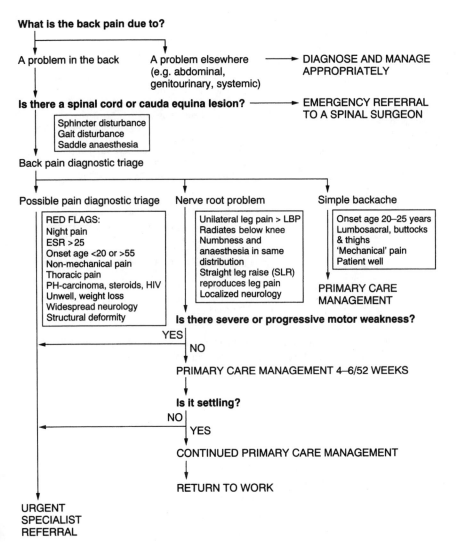

Figure 5.3   Diagnostic triage of a patient presenting with low back pain with or without sciatica. (Adapted from Clinical Standards Advisory Group 1994 *Back Pain*, HMSO, London)

SIMPLE BACKACHE

Onset generally age 20–55 years
Lumbosacral region, buttocks and thighs
Pain 'mechanical' in nature
 – varies with physical activity
 – varies with time
Patient well
Prognosis good
 – 90% recover from acute attack
   in 6 weeks

RED FLAGS

Possible serious spinal pathology:

Age of onset <25 or >55 years
Violent trauma: e.g. fall from a height, RTA
Constant, progressive, non-mechanical pain
Night pain
Thoracic pain
Past medical history – carcinoma
Systemic steroids
Drug abuse, HIV
Systemically unwell
Weight loss
Persisting severe restriction of lumbar
flexion
Widespread neurology
Structural deformity
ESR >25
Consider MRI scan/referral

NERVE ROOT PAIN

Unilateral leg pain > back pain
Pain generally radiates to below knee
Numbness and paraesthesia in the same
distribution
Nerve irritation signs
 – reduced straight leg raise which
   reproduces leg pain
Motor, sensory or reflex change
 – limited to one nerve root
Prognosis good
 – 90% recover from acute attack
   within 6 weeks

CAUDA EQUINA SYNDROME/ WIDESPREAD NEUROLOGICAL DISORDER

Difficulty with micturition
Loss of anal spincter tone or faecal
incontinence
Saddle anaesthesia about the anus, perineum
or genitals
Widespread (>one nerve root) or progressive
motor weakness in the legs or gait disturbance
Bilateral positive sciatic stretch test

INFLAMMATORY DISORDERS

Ankylosing spondylitis and related disorders
Gradual onset
Marked morning stiffness
Persisting limitation of spinal movements in all
directions
Peripheral joint involvement
Iritis, skin rashes (psoriasis), colitis, urethral
discharge
Family history

Figure 5.4 Diagnostic indicators for simple backache, nerve root pain, red flags, cauda equina syndrome and inflammatory disorders. (Adapted from Clinical Standards Advisory Group 1994 *Back Pain*, HMSO, London)

Inappropriate signs

Waddell has described various inappropriate signs, and if patients exhibit these signs, it is suggested there may be some overlay and exaggeration of their symptoms. These include widespread tenderness in the spine, non-anatomical weakness, jerky movements, non-anatomical sensory disturbance, pain in the lumbar spine or in the legs felt on axial compression along the spine, and reduced straight-leg raising while remaining able to sit on the examination couch with the knee extended and the hip fully flexed. However, these are only pointers to exaggerated behaviour and are more commonly associated with distress.

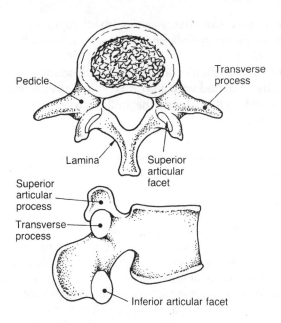

Figure 5.5 Anatomical features
of lumbar vertebra

COMMON SPINAL PROBLEMS

Mechanical low back pain

Between 60% and 90% of the population experience mechanical low back pain
at some time in their lives. It often follows an episode of heavy lifting or an
injury to the back. Fortunately, more than 90% of these patients have resolution
of their back pain within 6 weeks of the onset. Typically they are pain-free at
rest, with activity-induced pain. Up to 3 days of bed rest may be useful, but
thereafter physiotherapy and gradual return to activity are the main treatments
in the early stages. Patients with mechanical back pain should only be referred
to hospital if their symptoms continue for more than 6 weeks, and if the symptoms are severe enough to interfere significantly with day-to-day activities or
if the patient is unable to work. Invasive treatments are not usually indicated
unless the patient has had significant pain for up to a year.

It is important to differentiate mechanical back pain from back pain due to
infection or malignancy, where rest pain and night pain occur more commonly.

Disc prolapse

Disc prolapse is common in individuals between the ages of 20 and 60 years.
Occasionally this follows an acute incident, but usually the onset is gradual,
although there may be precipitating factors. Patients present initially with back
pain followed after 2–4 weeks by nerve root pain radiating down the leg into
the calf and the foot. Fortunately 90% of individuals with a disc prolapse will
have resolution of their symptoms in the first 6 weeks. Three days of bed rest
may help initially, as can early physiotherapy. Individuals with disc prolapse

commonly present with minor sensory disturbances and with alteration of the reflexes in the lower limbs. These are not specific indications for referral, but do help in establishing the exact diagnosis.

The patients usually present with back pain or occasionally with sciatic scoliosis. Straight leg raising is usually restricted with a positive sciatic stretch test on straight leg raising, with pain felt in the calf and the ankle or foot.

Indications for hospital referral are:

1. severe uncontrollable pain
2. symptoms which persist more than 6 weeks and are not improving
3. cauda equina symptoms of urinary and bowel symptoms (emergency referral)
4. weakness in the legs.

Sciatica is usually a self-limiting disease, and treatment is mainly helpful to accelerate recovery. This is particularly true of sciatica caused by disc prolapse. Surgery should only be considered where there is significant neurological dysfunction, or where pain is not resolving at 6 weeks.

If conservative treatment has not been successful, percutaneous nucleotomy has a success rate of about 60%. Discectomy and decompression of the nerve root is successful in 80–90% of cases. Where symptoms are mild or the patient is not suitable for surgery, epidural steroid injection may resolve the symptoms in a proportion of patients.

Scoliosis

Scoliosis usually presents in childhood. Occasionally elderly patients do present with a degenerative type of scoliosis which may give rise to symptoms of spinal instability or even spinal stenosis.

Scoliosis is a relatively common condition, with 10% of children having a slight scoliosis. However, scoliosis requiring surgery is only present in 2 in 1000 children. The three main types are neurogenic scoliosis, congenital scoliosis of a structural type and, most common in the UK, idiopathic scoliosis. Neurogenic and structural type scoliosis usually present at a young age, and an early referral for a specialist opinion is indicated. Idiopathic scoliosis may present early (10% of cases), but the vast majority (90%) present during the adolescent years as adolescent idiopathic scoliosis. These patients need to be reassured that it is simply a cosmetic condition, providing there is no obvious underlying cause for the scoliosis. Any child with a significant scoliosis should be referred for a specialist opinion.

Spinal stenosis

This condition typically presents in individuals over 60 years of age. It is usually associated with degenerative changes in the lumbar spine, and a combination of loss of disc space, new bone formation due to osteophytes and infolding at the ligamentum flavum compress the nerve roots laterally at the

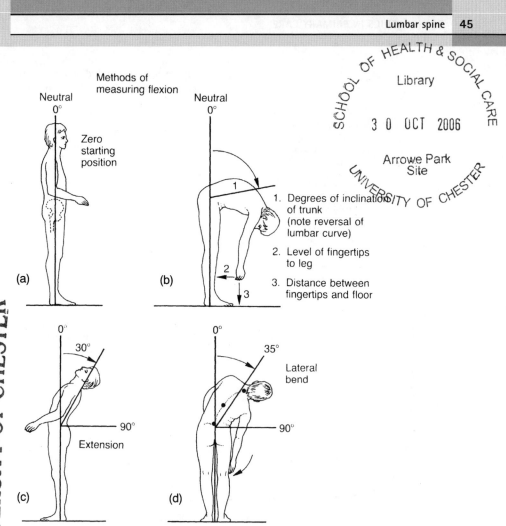

Methods of measuring flexion

Neutral 0°

Neutral 0°

Zero starting position

1. Degrees of inclination of trunk (note reversal of lumbar curve)

2. Level of fingertips to leg

3. Distance between fingertips and floor

(a)

(b)

0°

30°

90°

Extension

(c)

0°

35°

Lateral bend

90°

(d)

Figure 5.6   (a) Flexion – zero starting point; (b) methods of measuring flexion; (c) extension; (d) lateral bend

beginning but ultimately may cause a central type of stenosis. At worst, this may cause symptoms of cauda equina compression. The symptoms are usually of insidious onset and increase gradually over a number of years. There is not usually any associated injury. Half of patients present with a history of back pain. The typical symptoms are of pain in the leg with or without weakness or numbness, which usually occurs on walking. The patients are typically better walking uphill than downhill and are better cycling than walking, as flexion of the spine tends to have the effect of partially decompressing the nerve roots. Occasionally the patient will present with bowel or urinary symptoms but in most the symptoms are of gradual onset.

Physiotherapy with flexion exercises may be helpful for this condition. Epidurals are occasionally helpful although the success rate is probably less than 20%.

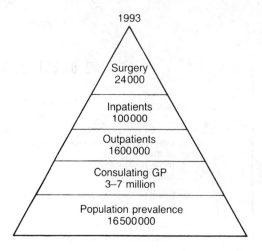

Figure 5.7 Estimated annual health care for back pain in 1993 (number of cases)

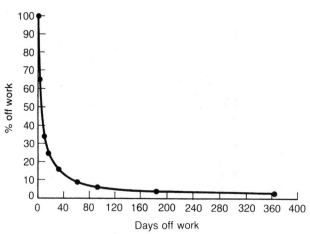

Figure 5.8 Duration of work loss with back pain; over 90% of sufferers will return to work within 50 days

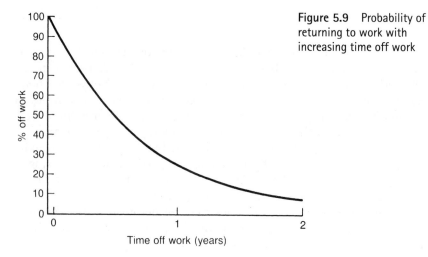

Figure 5.9 Probability of returning to work with increasing time off work

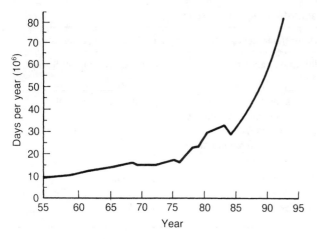

Figure 5.10   Total British Sickness and Invalidity Benefit for incapacities increased between 1955 and 1993

Emergency and urgent referrals

The initial diagnostic triage will identify the small number of patients requiring urgent and emergency referral to a hospital specialist. Guidelines for emergency and urgent referrals are set out below.

Emergency referral:
Diagnosis:	Acute spinal cord damage/acute cauda equina syndrome/widespread neurological disorder
Action:	Emergency referral to a specialist with experience in spinal surgery immediately

Urgent referrals (within a few weeks):
Diagnosis:	Possible serious spinal pathology
Action:	Urgent referral for specialist investigation, generally to an orthopaedic surgeon or a rheumatologist, depending on local availability
Diagnosis:	Possible acute inflammatory disorders
Action:	Urgent referral to a rheumatologist
Diagnosis:	Nerve root problem
Action:	Should generally be dealt with initially by the GP, providing there is no major progressive motor weakness. Early referral may be required for additional acute pain control. If it is not resolving satisfactorily after 6 weeks, the patient should be referred urgently for appropriate specialist assessment and investigation

Figure 5.11   Indications for emergency and urgent referral. (Adapted from Clinical Standards Advisory Group 1994 *Back Pain*, HMSO, London)

Surgery is indicated in patients who have not responded to conservative measures. Patients with significant symptoms which either affect their day-to-day life or prevent them working should be referred. The success rate for this type of surgery is approximately 70%.

Spinal infection

Spinal infection is rare and patients present with a constant unremitting back pain, particularly at night. The pain often keeps them awake. They may complain of a temperature or rigors. Spasm is often present in the paraspinal

Table 5.2   Summary of diagnostic triage and referral

Possible serious spinal pathology	Urgent/emergency referral for specialist investigation	
	Initial management	If not resolving by 4–6 weeks
Nerve root problem	General practitioner ? Refer for acute pain control ? Physiotherapy ?? Osteopathy/chiropractic	Urgent surgical referral
Simple backache	General practitioner ? Physiotherapy ? Osteopathy/chiropractic ?? Refer for acute pain control	Psychological and vocational assessment Active rehabilitation for return to work

Table 5.3   Comparative clinical features of spinal stenosis, peripheral vascular disease and disc disease

Feature	Spinal stenosis	Disc prolapse	Peripheral vascular disease
Reduced straight leg raise	Rarely	Usually	No
Neurological deficit	Sometimes	Often	No
Leg pain on walking	Yes	Usually	Yes
Leg pain on sitting	No	Yes	No
Pain relief on standing still	No	No	Yes
Pain relief on sitting	Yes	No	Yes
Numbness/paraesthesiae	Yes	Yes	Sometimes

muscles and patients are usually tender at the site of the infection, although clinical signs are notoriously unreliable. This condition is more common in individuals with diabetes, and also in the immunosuppressed or those who have had cardiac or urinary catheterization. Tuberculosis is relatively common especially in the Indian community and in immigrants. Urgent referral is indicated, as early treatment with intravenous antibiotics is usually successful.

Spinal tumours

Ninety per cent of spinal tumours are due to secondary deposits, and therefore a majority of the patients presenting with this will have a history of a previous malignant tumour. Like infection, the symptoms are usually of gradually increasing pain which is constant in nature, and may keep the patient awake at night. There may be neurological signs if there is compression on the spinal cord or the nerve roots. Plain X-ray is useful in assisting diagnosis, but early referral is recommended. MRI is the preferred way of establishing a diagnosis. Most of these patients will respond to radiotherapy, but occasionally surgery is necessary either for compressive symptoms or rarely for unresolved pain.

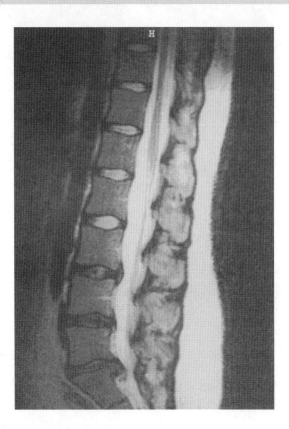

Figure 5.12   MRI showing a prolapsed L5/S1 disc

IMAGING TECHNIQUES

Indications for radiography

MRI scan is the investigation of choice in spinal disorders, and has largely replaced plain X-ray in the UK. MRI is very sensitive for almost all spinal conditions. However, the results should be interpreted with care. Twenty per cent of asymptomatic individuals have disc prolapse, and with increasing age nearly everyone has evidence of degenerative changes.

X-rays are of limited value in the diagnosis and management of most patients with spinal disorders. It has been estimated that approximately 1% of X-rays change the management of these patients. X-rays may be of value in diagnosis in some cases of mechanical disorder, such as spondylolisthesis and in the diagnosis of and management of spinal deformities such as kyphosis or scoliosis. Plain X-rays are of no value in the diagnosis of disorders such as disc prolapse and spinal stenosis.

Where MRI is not available, X-rays may be helpful in the diagnosis of infection or tumour.

Chapter 6

Hip

Richard de Steiger

- Referral for hip replacement surgery should be based on individual disability and levels of pain – old age is not a contraindication.
- Loosening of a hip joint replacement occurs in approximately 5% of patients at 10 years.
- Trochanteric bursitis responds well to steroid injections.
- Septic arthritis of the hip may present insidiously.

PRESENTING SYMPTOMS

Adult hip problems usually present with pain in the groin and thigh. Symptoms may radiate to the knee. Stiffness and leg shortening may also be a feature, particularly in arthritis, and will usually cause an abnormal gait. A limp is a common feature of hip pathology.

PHYSICAL EXAMINATION

Hip examination should include a brief assessment of gait though abnormalities may only be apparent if the patient has walked for some distance. An antalgic gait is one in which the patient, because of pain, spends less time on the affected side during the stance phase of gait. Leg length should be checked, especially to note if there is any apparent discrepancy because of fixed hip deformity. A passive range of motion is next carried out. Often internal rotation is the first movement lost. A normal range of motion for a hip joint is 120 degrees of flexion, 45 degrees of abduction, 30 degrees of adduction, 45 degrees of external rotation and 45 degrees of internal rotation. As lumbar spine problems can commonly present as pain around the hip joint, examination of the lumbar spine and, if appropriate, a lower limb neurological examination should be performed.

Table 6.1   Common causes of hip pain in different age groups

| Age group | Cause | | |
	Intra–articular	Periarticular	Referred
Childhood (2–10 years)	Developmental dislocation of the hip Perthes' disease Irritable hip Rickets	Osteomyelitis	Abdominal
Adolescence (10–18 years)	Slipped upper femoral epiphysis Torn labrum	Trochanteric bursitis Snapping hip Osteomyelitis Tumours	Abdominal Lumbar spine
Early adulthood (18–30 years)	Inflammatory arthritis Torn labrum	Bursitis	Abdominal Lumbar spine
Adulthood (30–50 years)	Osteoarthritis Inflammatory arthritis Osteonecrosis Transient osteoporosis	Bursitis	Abdominal Lumbar spine
Old age (>50 years)	Osteoarthritis Inflammatory arthritis		Abdominal Lumbar spine

Table 6.2   Normal range of movement: hip

Flexion	0–120 degrees
Extension	0–30 degrees
Abduction	0–45 degrees
Adduction	0–30 degrees
Internal rotation	0–45 degrees
External rotation	0–45 degrees

COMMON HIP PROBLEMS

Arthritis

Almost any cause of systemic arthritis can involve the hip joint, but by far the most common is osteoarthritis (OA). Radiographic signs of hip OA affect between 5% and 10% of the population to some degree. Although small joints are most commonly affected in rheumatoid arthritis, the hip may be involved in progressive disease. The various inflammatory arthropathies and other metabolic disorders may also involve the hip.

The usual first symptom of early hip arthritis is dull pain in the groin radiating to the buttock, lateral thigh and often to the knee. The pain is exacerbated by movement, in particular standing up from a seated position, and is worse at the end of a long day. Rest improves the pain in the early stages, but as the disorder progresses, patients have pain even when resting or in bed. Patients begin to limp, especially after walking for a distance, and commonly complain that they are unable to perform simple tasks such as putting on shoes and socks or having a bath.

The earliest clinical examination finding is loss of internal rotation. This is followed by reduced flexion and abduction. The back should also be examined as patients with OA have an increased incidence of degenerative lumbar spine disease. The classic X-ray of findings of OA are joint space narrowing, osteophytes, subchondral sclerosis and cyst formation, and these are present in varying degrees according to the severity.

Management of this widespread condition is based on treating the patient's main symptom, which is pain, and the secondary symptom, which is disability. Patients initially need some education about the natural history of OA as many think they are doomed to a progressive downhill course, leaving them severely disabled. This is rarely the case, and the symptoms from hip OA tend to wax and wane and do not always irretrievably worsen.

Many people wish to know what they can and cannot do in terms of daily activities and sporting pursuits. As a general rule, the more vigorous and demanding a sport the more likely the patient is to suffer from hip pain during or after the event. Patients can be advised to be sensible about pursuing activities and there is certainly no reason for them to stop. Activities such as walking, swimming, bicycle riding and gardening can all be continued without undue risk to the hip. If the patient knows that a particular activity is likely to cause pain, then it is perfectly sensible for them to take analgesics before undertaking the activity.

For the pain, simple analgesics are the first line of therapy. There is little evidence that NSAIDs alter the course of osteoarthritis. Though they may provide some initial pain relief, they are probably inappropriate for long-term management. Maintaining a range of movement in any arthritic joint is important, and simple exercises, swimming and, in more severe cases, referral to a physiotherapist for hydrotherapy treatment, may help.

A stick, used in the *opposite* hand to the diseased hip, will help unload the force through the affected joint and improve gait. A simple shoe insole may also help some people. Although weight loss for those who are overweight is sensible advice it is often difficult to achieve. Its main benefit may be in minimizing the small risks involved in surgery.

The decision to refer for surgery is based largely on the level of the pain and the disabilities the patient describes. Loss of independence, especially in elderly people, or an inability to work in younger people are very relevant. Total joint replacement has revolutionized the treatment of hip osteoarthritis, but osteotomy and, in some cases, arthrodesis of the hip should still be considered in the younger patient. Intracapsular hip joint injection may occasionally help, but its main use is diagnostic when there is doubt as to whether the pain is lumbar or hip related. Following hip replacement, patients usually require 7–10 days in hospital and are discharged on crutches or a stick.

As a result of the large number of primary hip replacements performed, many artificial joints are now becoming loose, resulting in the need for revision hip replacement. This is an increasing problem and as a general rule any patient who has recurrence of pain in a previously replaced joint should be sent for specialist advice. Plain radiographs are often difficult to interpret.

Avascular necrosis

Avascular necrosis, or osteonecrosis, is a disorder which may affect several bones, but commonly occurs in the hip joints. As the name implies, there is an

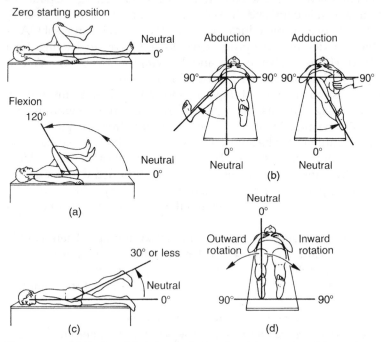

Figure 6.1 (a) Flexion; (b) abduction/adduction; (c) extension; (d) rotation

Table 6.3 Indications for hip replacement surgery

Pain	This is the principal indication for surgery. Pain that occurs at rest and at night, severe pain on movement and pain poorly controlled with analgesic medication are also strong indicators
Activities of daily living	If the restricted movement and pain caused by the arthritis are significantly affecting ability to walk, dress, wash, etc. then this is a relative indication for total hip replacement
Age	Because joint replacements have a limited survival, surgery under the age of 55 or 60 has to be considered especially carefully

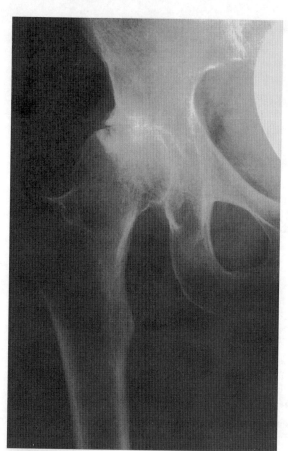

Figure 6.2 X-ray of an osteoarthritic hip

Figure 6.3 X-ray of a total hip replacement

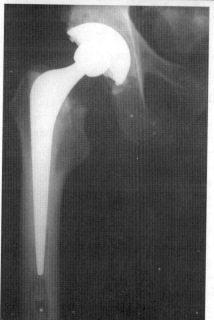

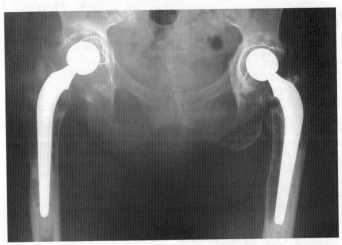

Figure 6.4   X-ray of a loose total hip replacement

Table 6.4   Indications of problems with a hip replacement

Pain	Any significant and sustained increase in pain around a joint replacement should be investigated. If in doubt refer. Some patients have a persistent ache around the hip and thigh, even in an otherwise successful joint replacement
Loss of movement	Artificial joints are often stiff but a sudden loss of movement should be investigated with a radiograph
Leg-length discrepancy	Some patients will have leg-length discrepancy from the outset. This can usually be corrected with a heel raise
Dislocation	Occasionally hip replacements dislocate. This is invariably a painful and acute event and requires emergency referral. The leg will usually appear short and externally rotated
Fracture	Fractures can occur around artificial joints, particularly if they are loose. They usually present acutely with severe pain and loss of function. Emergency referral is indicated
Loosening	Aseptic loosening of joint replacements occurs in about 5% of cases at 10 years. It will usually present with gradual onset of pain and should be investigated with an X-ray. If loosening is present then refer
Infection	Deep infection is rare after joint replacements (<3%). It will usually present with pain. Sometimes local signs are present. Rarely the patient may be systemically unwell; emergency referral is indicated in these situations
DVT and pulmonary embolus	DVT is common after lower limb joint replacement. Isolated calf vein thromboses can be treated conservatively but thrombi extending higher than the knee are probably best treated with heparin and 3 months warfarin. Deaths from pulmonary emboli are rare (<1%)

interruption to the blood supply of the femoral head. This classically results in a pathological, crescent-shaped fracture of the femoral head. Patients at risk of developing this condition include immunosuppressed patients with renal transplants, patients receiving steroid therapy, patients who have sickle cell disease, deep-sea divers and patients who overuse alcohol. The commonest background, however, is a delayed presentation following trauma to the femoral head or neck. Typically the patient presents with a dull pain in the groin which is usually exacerbated by weight bearing. The condition is frequently bilateral in the non-traumatic group but presenting at different times. Radiographs may be entirely normal in the early stages, but by the time the patient has moderate symptoms they show a subchondral fracture of the femoral head. MRI will show medullary changes of avascular necrosis before any radiographic changes are apparent.

Early referral is appropriate. The outcome largely depends on the extent of involvement of the femoral head. Many treatments have been proposed for relief of pain, but these do not always alter the long-term outcome. One option is core decompression by drilling a hole up through the femoral neck. In selected cases, osteotomy to replace an area of dead bone with viable articular cartilage or bone grafting into the femoral head may help.

Acetabular dysplasia

Acetabular dysplasia is a condition in which the acetabulum fails to fully develop. The adult's acetabulum in this condition is shallow, leaving the anterolateral part of the femoral head uncovered. People, usually women, present in their third to fourth decade with hip pain after exercise or a busy day. The pain generally disappears with rest but may persist. Examination of the hip reveals a full range of movement, which is painful only in the extremes of flexion and internal rotation. Sometimes patients with a tear of the acetabular labrum complain of a feeling of instability. This feeling can often be reproduced during the examination of extension and external rotation.

X-rays reveal a shallow acetabulum with femoral head subluxation of a varying degree. Early arthrosis may be present. This condition, if left untreated, may lead to increasing pain and eventually arthritis of the hip joint, especially if there is an incongruity between the femoral head and the acetabulum.

Referral is indicated to discuss the natural history of the disorder and to plan treatment options. To relieve symptoms and prevent the onset of arthritis, some form of cover of the femoral head is required. This can be achieved by introducing a simple shelf of bone over the capsule or by more complex periacetabular osteotomies. Unfortunately, in some instances the joint is incongruent and this leads to secondary OA and the need for joint replacement.

Infection

Although this is a relatively uncommon problem in the adult hip, it is important to diagnose because failure to treat may have disastrous effects on the hip joint itself. Septic arthritis of the hip is more common in childhood but over the last few decades the incidence in adults has increased. Bacteria can infect the hip joint through three mechanisms: haematogenous spread, spread from a nearby focus, or direct inoculation at the time of surgery or trauma. As with other forms of infection, certain groups of patients are at risk, including those with chronic diseases such as diabetes, renal failure, rheumatoid arthritis, immunocompromised patients, especially if on systemic steroids, and patients who are malnourished. The commonest organisms involved are *Staphylococcus aureus* and streptococcus. Tuberculosis, however, must always be considered. The onset may sometimes be insidious. Pain is the usual initial symptom though the patient may complain of fever or chills. The hip is extremely irritable on examination and sometimes cannot be moved. A raised temperature is not always found.

Urgent referral for treatment is essential, for confirmation of the diagnosis by ultrasound-guided aspiration or athrotomy. Treatment includes a washout of the joint, followed by appropriate intravenous antibiotics, guided by the microbiological findings. If treatment is prompt the joint can usually be salvaged, but, in delayed cases, cartilage destruction and secondary OA may result.

Tumours

Primary bone tumours affecting the hip area are rare, but metastatic spread of tumour to the proximal femur and acetabulum are much more common. Carcinoma of the breast, colon, prostate and thyroid are the main neoplasms to metastasize to the hip. Sometimes, in fact, the presenting symptom for an undiagnosed primary is pain around the hip.

In any patient with a previous malignancy who presents with vague deep-seated hip pain, metastatic spread to bone should be considered. Plain X-rays usually show up any significant lesions but a bone scan is more sensitive in detecting smaller tumours. Patients should be treated surgically if severe pain cannot be controlled or the bone is likely to fracture. A cemented joint replacement or hemiarthroplasty may provide relief from pain and give a patient mobility. Operations are appropriate even though the patient's expectation of life has been shortened. These patients are at slightly higher risk of wound breakdown from deep infection, especially if there has been prior radiotherapy to the involved area.

When treating a young adult for a presumed soft tissue problem around the hip which does not improve or worsens, beware of deep, continuous pain, especially if unrelated to activity and occurring at night. Osteosarcoma, though rare, must be borne in mind and investigated by requesting an X-ray.

SOFT TISSUE PROBLEMS ABOUT THE HIP

Underlying muscle strains and tendonitis

Muscle strains about the hip usually follow sudden violent exercise, while tendonitis usually occurs after repetitive chronic overuse. Common sites involved around the hip are the ischial tuberosity, at the origin of the hamstring muscles and along the edge of the pubic ramus at the origin of the adductor longus muscle. The pain is usually localized to these areas but may radiate down the thigh.

If the strain follows an acute injury cold packs and compression to restrict bleeding may help. In the more chronic conditions NSAIDs, heat and ultrasound can all be of benefit. Injection at the tender site with local anaesthetic and cortisone can be tried in resistant cases.

Trochanteric bursitis

This condition is an inflammation of the bursa over the greater trochanter. It is most commonly seen in runners. Patients complain of a deep aching, located on or just behind the greater trochanter, and often are unable to sleep on the affected side. There is well-localized tenderness to palpation over the trochanter. This is usually a self-limiting condition and can be treated initially with heat and topical non-steroidal creams. If the condition persists, a local anaesthetic and steroid injection into the most tender spot will usually resolve the symptoms. This is a safe procedure to perform using 40 mg of steroid preparation and 2–5 ml of marcaine.

Gluteus medius tendonitis can present with pain around the lateral aspect of the hip and, in some cases can be difficult to distinguish from trochanteric bursitis. Anti-inflammatory medication and stretching exercises can help.

Snapping hip syndrome

This is a condition usually found in dancers and adolescent girls, whereby the iliotibial band rubs or snaps over the greater trochanter. Patients complain of a click or snap when they flex and rotate their hip. The condition occurs intermittently and is uncomfortable rather than painful. Reassurance is the key: nothing seriously is wrong, and most patients ignore the symptom. Occasionally, in some people with persistent or painful symptoms, lengthening the iliotibial band may help.

Chapter 7

Knee

C. L. M. H. Gibbons

- Anterior knee pain in adolescents is common, often bilateral and treatment is conservative.
- X-ray examination of the knee is often normal in the younger patient.
- Degenerative meniscal tears characteristically cause mechanical and nocturnal knee pain.
- Anterior cruciate rupture is the most common knee injury caused while skiing.
- Steroid injections of the knee should be intra-articular.

PRESENTING SYMPTOMS

Pain

1. Pain may be localized or diffuse. It is useful to ask the patient to indicate the site of the pain by drawing or pointing to the area of discomfort.
2. Localized pain is usually highly significant, whereas diffuse pain is less likely to signify surgical pathology.

Swelling

1. Immediate swelling, particularly after an injury, is suggestive of a haemarthrosis such as following a cruciate ligament rupture.
2. Gradual swelling, e.g. overnight, is more suggestive of a reactive effusion such as with a meniscal tear.
3. Recurrent swelling in the absence of trauma is more indicative of chronic disease such as degenerative osteoarthritis or an inflammatory arthropathy.

Locking

Locking is a term which describes the inability to fully extend the knee. This implies there is a mechanical block of the full range of movement due to an intra-articular cause such as a torn meniscus or loose body.

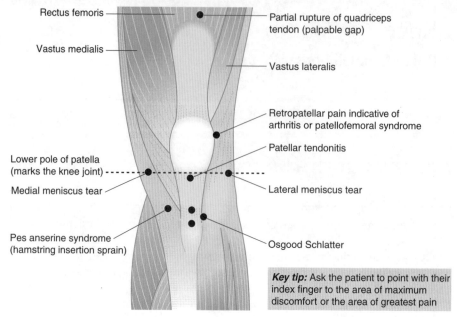

Figure 7.1   Localized pain and knee disorder

Pseudolocking

Clicking or catching of the knee usually provoked with stair descent or ascent is suggestive of patellofemoral articular damage.

Giving way

This is a mechanical event which occurs when the weight-bearing knee in slight flexion is put under sudden extra stress such as in running or 'cutting' to the side. This is the hallmark symptom of a cruciate ligament rupture.

PHYSICAL EXAMINATION

Look

The patient should be examined walking, standing and lying. With the patient standing upright the degree of overall alignment from in front (knee varus and valgus) and from the side (hyperextension and flexion deformity of the knee) are measured. On lying, thigh, knee and leg are examined in sequence.

Quadriceps wasting occurs quickly with disuse and is best assessed by comparing active contraction (ask the patient to press the knee firmly into the couch) and measurement with a tape at a fixed point above the patella.

Table 7.1   Common causes of knee pain in different age groups

Age group	Cause Intra-articular	Periarticular	Referred
Childhood (2–10 years)	Juvenile arthritis Osteochondritis dissecans Infection Torn discoid meniscus	Osteomyelitis	Perthes' disease Irritable hip
Adolescence (10–18 years)	Osteochondritis dissecans Torn meniscus Anterior knee pain syndrome Patellar instability	Osgood–Schlatter disease Sinding–Larsen– Johansson syndrome Osteomyelitis Bone tumours	Slipped upper femoral epiphysis
Early adulthood (18–30 years)	Torn meniscus Patellar instability Anterior knee pain syndrome Inflammatory arthritis	Ligament injuries Bursitis	
Adulthood (30–50 years)	Degenerate meniscal tears Osteoarthritis Inflammatory arthritis	Bursitis	Osteoarthritis of hip Spinal disorders
Old age (>50 years)	Osteoarthritis Inflammatory arthritis	Bursitis	Osteoarthritis of hip Spinal disorders

The presence of surgical scars and swellings around the knee should be noted. Localized swelling is suggestive of extra-articular pathology and the joint line and nature of the swelling (cystic or solid) should be carefully assessed. Symmetrical and generalized swelling of the knee is more indicative of intra-articular pathology where the swelling is seen above and either side of the patella.

Feel

Palpation can often be useful, particularly if there is local tenderness, suggesting focal pathology, rather than diffuse tenderness which suggests generalized inflammation. A large, tense swelling indicates a haemarthrosis or infection, whereas a lax swelling is usually secondary to a reactive effusion associated with synovitis.

The knee should be first examined flat in extension and the presence of an effusion assessed by stroking the fluid from the suprapatellar pouch into the

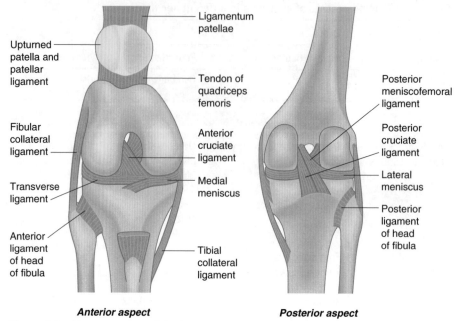

Figure 7.2   Ligaments around the knee

parapatellar gutters. Any evidence of synovial thickening should be noted. A clinically obvious effusion is always significant. With the knee then flexed to 90 degrees, a popliteal swelling or cyst may be palpated at the back of the knee and this is usually more prominent in extension.

With the knee flexed at 90 degrees, the joint line should be carefully examined for localized pain. Pain is commonly localized to the posterior medial joint line with a degenerative meniscal tear or an acute medial meniscal injury. Again, ask the patient to point to the area of maximum discomfort.

Move

Examination of the movement of the joint should begin by lifting both heels. Fixed flexion or extension deformities will be easily seen. A 'springy block' to full extension suggests significant meniscal pathology, whereas a solid block usually suggests longstanding pathology such as osteoarthrosis.

The active (the patient moves the limb), followed by the passive (you move the limb), range of movement should then be documented. Range of motion is assessed, looking in particular for loss of motion and for how smoothly the movement takes place. The extensor mechanism should be palpated and, in particular, any irritability and/or crepitus noted. The patient should be assessed sitting on the edge of the couch actively flexing and extending the knee. With a hand on the patella any lateral subluxation is tested (apprehension test), and is more florid with the knee in full extension.

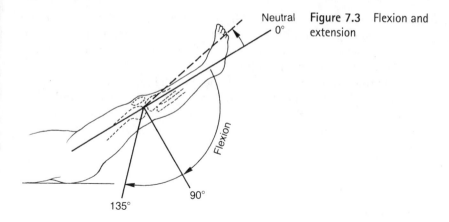

Neutral   **Figure 7.3**   Flexion and
0°   extension

Flexion

90°

135°

Table 7.2   Normal range of movement: knee

Flexion	0–135 degrees

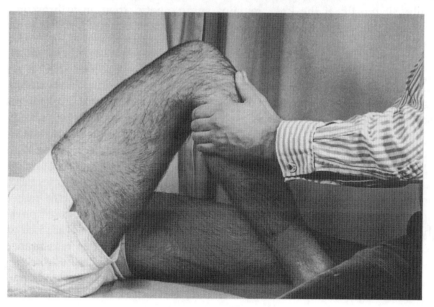

Figure 7.4   Testing for knee instability – the anterior draw test

Special tests

Specific tests should then be undertaken:

McMurray (meniscal provocation test): internal/external rotation of the flexed knee, looking for pain and clicking over the medial/lateral jointline (assessment of pathology in the posterior horn of the meniscus).

Lachman: attempted anterior draw of the tibia on the femur in 20 degrees flexion (the most sensitive test for damage of the anterior cruciate).

Anterior draw: As Lachman, but attempted at 90 degrees flexion. With the knee flexed to 90 degrees and the hamstrings relaxed, attempt to draw the tibia forwards. In anterior cruciate deficiency there will be excessive forward movement normally with no end point.

To complete this examination an assessment of the hip joint and the spine should be undertaken to exclude referred pain. In addition a neurological examination of the lower limbs and an assessment of peripheral pulses should be carried out to exclude a spinal, vascular or neurological cause of referred knee pain.

COMMON KNEE PROBLEMS

Discoid meniscus

This presents in young patients (2–10 years old), and may be bilateral with clicking, catching usually of the lateral joint line and chronic symptomatology. Examination may reveal a minor flexion contracture with joint line tenderness. Investigation with radiographs may reveal a widened joint space, and MRI is usually diagnostic. If the knee remains symptomatic, then an arthroscopic examination may be indicated. Menisectomy is usually only undertaken if the meniscus is torn.

Patellofemoral syndrome

This syndrome most often affects adolescents, usually girls with spontaneous onset, and is often bilateral with recurrent anterior knee pain. Often the history of symptoms goes back 1 or 2 years with pain aggravated by climbing stairs, changing gears in a car, prolonged sitting ('cinema knee') and wearing high heels. Examination often reveals retropatellar crepitus and irritability. Quadriceps weakness may be present and the hamstrings are sometimes tight, otherwise examination is usually unremarkable. Investigation with radiographs is usually not indicated. MRI is normally reserved for after failed physiotherapy treatment and for reassurance. Conservative treatment is advised as this is generally a self-limiting problem. Detailed explanation and reassurance is required. NSAIDs and splintage in the acute phase can be helpful. Bracing may be added as the patient improves. Physiotherapy is very important, and the patient may need repeat sessions. Surgery is not indicated and is contemplated only after failure of prolonged conservative treatment. Arthroscopy is performed to exclude other causes and sometimes arthroscopic lateral release is advised, but this procedure is not without complications. Patella realignment is occasionally undertaken but it may not be curative and is associated with significant early and late complications.

Patellar instability

Patellar instability or malalignment is common in adolescence, often bilateral affecting girls, and significant if there has been a documented episode of patella dislocation or subluxation. Patella alta, genu valgum, external tibial torsion and persistent femoral anteversion are all causes of this problem. Acute dislocation may be associated with osteochondral fracture. Patellar subluxation is more common than complete dislocation.

Clinical examination may be normal and there are a number of subtle signs. Examine carefully for quadriceps wasting and patellar irritability with and without crepitus. Instability is associated with ligament laxity and valgus knee deformity and enquire about double jointedness. The apprehension sign (patient apprehension as the examiner attempts to laterally displace the patella) and tenderness over the medial border of the patella with an acute presentation are particularly significant. Plain X-rays, including true lateral and skyline views, are useful in the assessment of patellar abnormality, trochlea dysplasia and subluxation. Dynamic MRI of the patella tracking in the femoral groove (trochlea) will predict which patients may require surgery, and is particularly useful in those who have had episodes of subluxation or dislocation.

Initial conservative treatment is usually advised, which includes supervised and home programmes of exercise and rehabilitation with bracing. Surgical arthroscopic lateral release has a less than 60% success rate. Where there is clear evidence of patella instability in the dynamic studies, tibial tubercle realignment (Emslie–Trillat operation), although more invasive, will guarantee a good outcome in the majority of cases.

Meniscal tear

This is a common sports-related injury (soccer, athletics, rugby). It may be an acute event usually brought on by twisting on the weight-bearing leg. The patient may complain of clicking, catching and locking. Swelling is unusual. In the sportsman a meniscal tear is usually a longitudinal or 'parrot-beak' and may be associated with an anterior cruciate ligament (ACL) injury. In the older patient with a more indolent history where there may not be a precipitating event, a horizontal radial tear (degenerate variety) is more common. On examination, quadriceps muscle wasting is almost an invariable finding. A joint effusion (delayed onset) with joint line tenderness and a positive McMurray's test is evident. A minor flexion deformity with a springy block to extension (if large displaced tear) is very significant. Radiographs are rarely helpful, but MRI will confirm the diagnosis. Arthroscopic meniscectomy is the treatment of choice. Longitudinal, peripheral tears in the younger patient are repaired with sutures if possible.

Anterior cruciate rupture

This affects the young adult involved in a sports-related injury. Usually the trauma is as a result of a non-contact injury with the patient falling to the floor. Often there is no contact and immediate swelling is a very common presentation. The patient may describe a 'pop' or 'crack'. The pain is usually intense and the injured person is often taken to casualty. The acute symptoms last

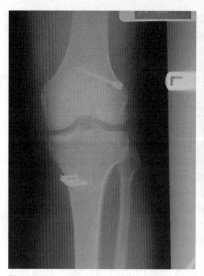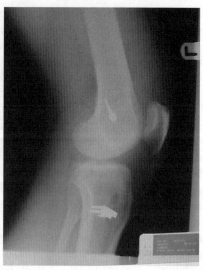

Figure 7.5   Anterior cruciate ligament reconstruction showing screw fixation of the bone tendon graft

a week or so, then settle. Once the acute phase is over the patient often complains of recurrent giving way, saying that their knee feels unstable on returning to sport. Examination is often difficult immediately after the injury but a haemarthrosis may be present. A positive Lachman test is invariably present (AP draw at 20 degrees), whereas an anterior draw (AP draw at 90 degrees) may be difficult to elicit because of pain and spasm. There may be signs of a positive pivot shift test, indicating anterolateral rotatory instability. Signs of meniscal damage should also be sought by examining for joint line tenderness and a positive McMurray's test.

Radiographs may exclude bony injury in the very painful acute presentation, otherwise they are rarely helpful. MRI is very useful for assessing both cruciate ligaments and for associated meniscal damage. Conservative treatment includes proprioceptive hamstring rehabilitation and allows the acute injury to settle. Reconstruction is appropriate for younger sports patients or those patients who have functional symptoms despite conservative treatment.

Degenerative meniscal tear

This is seen in middle-aged patients with a fairly innocuous injury. Indeed, patients may not even remember a trauma episode. Chronic symptomatology with night pain is highly specific. Twisting or squatting down tend to exacerbate symptoms. Quadriceps wasting with a minor flexion deformity and joint line tenderness are very suggestive of significant 'surgical' pathology. X-rays may show minor osteoarthritis. MRI reveals the characteristic appearance of a tear. Arthroscopic partial meniscectomy is the treatment of choice if there are major signs of mechanical disruption or if an intra-articular steroid injection fails to settle symptoms.

Symptomatic loose body formation

This is an uncommon complaint. The patient may feel loose body within the knee ('knee mouse'). The patient is often symptom-free with acute episodes of sudden severe pain, catching, locking and swelling of the joint. A knee effusion with quadriceps wasting and a minor flexion deformity is usual. A palpable loose body (suprapatellar pouch or lateral gutter) will confirm the diagnosis. X-rays are often diagnostic with a true loose body seen and an intercondylar view to localize the loose body is often useful. Calcified loose bodies reported on X-ray are often anchored in the synovium and may be fixed. A loose body is often confused with the fabella which is a sesamoid bone and a normal finding on X-ray. Arthroscopic assessment and surgery with removal of the loose body usually results in the successful resolution of knee symptoms.

Early osteoarthritis

This is seen in middle-aged patients and there may be a previous history of injury or surgery such as an open medial meniscectomy. Pain and swelling are associated with exercise and activity. Pain is usually improved with rest and anti-inflammatory medication. Clinical examination confirms a mild quadriceps wasting with diffuse joint line tenderness and a minor flexion or varus contracture which is suggestive of degenerative pathology. Physiotherapy is helpful in early disease and intra-articular steroid injection with local anaesthetic is useful and may be repeated to control early symptomatic disease. Arthroscopy is reserved for recalcitrant cases and may give temporary syptomatic relief, particularly if there are mechanical symptoms.

Established osteoarthritis

This presents in middle to old age with chronic symptoms. Acute exacerbations usually settle quickly. There is pain and swelling with activity. An established flexion and varus or valgus deformity with reduced movement is commonly present. Irritability, crepitus with patella movement and secondary ligamentous laxity are encountered. A weight-bearing true lateral X-ray is usually very helpful and for patellofemoral OA, a skyline view is required. NSAID medication, physiotherapy, weight reduction, a walking stick and a home programme of rehabilitation exercises should be tried before considering surgery. Bracing the knee is often helpful if instability is a problem. Arthroscopic surgery is unpredictable, but can give dramatic relief. The role of arthroscopic abrasion chondroplasty is yet to be defined, but it may relieve mechanical symptoms. With radiographic and clinical end-stage disease, total knee replacement is very effective in relieving symptoms.

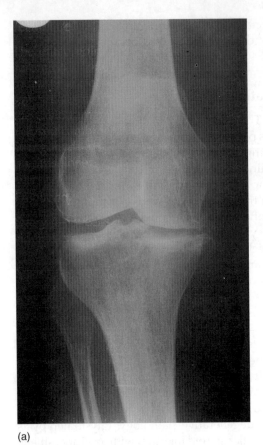

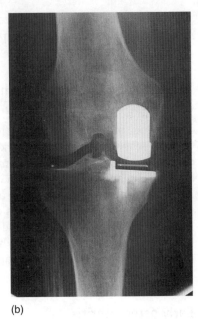

(b)

(a)

Figure 7.6 (a) Medial compartment osteoarthritis with (b) Oxford Unicompartmental knee replacement

Bursitis

Bursitis is a common problem due to inflammation of the bursae around the knee.

Prepatellar bursitis (housemaid's knee)

This is an occupational hazard in people who spend a great deal of time kneeling, such as carpet-layers, tilers and plumbers. Clinically there is a warm, tender, well-circumscribed, fluctuant lesion over the front of the patella, which may look infected but usually is not. Most lesions settle with rest and avoidance of kneeling. Occasionally aspiration is necessary and if this fails then surgical excision is only very rarely indicated.

Infrapatellar bursitis (parson's knee)

This fits the description of prepatellar bursitis, but with the swelling below the patella over the patella tendon.

Tendonitis

This presents with pain with or without localized swelling at the para-articular tendon insertions. This is usually a sports-related condition or an overuse injury.

Patellar tendonitis (jumper's knee)

This is a sports-related condition and symptoms are localized to the inferior pole of the patella and are exacerbated by activity, particularly climbing stairs, running or jumping. Pain and swelling over the inferior pole of the patella are often present. Most cases respond to rest and NSAIDs. In persistent cases, ultrasound- or MRI-guided injection of steroid and local anaesthetic is often curative, but occasionally, surgical decompression is necessary for recalcitrant cases.

Other common sites of tendonitis

Other relatively common sites of tendonitis of the knee are:

1. iliotibial band friction syndrome (runner's/cyclist's knee)
2. hamstring tendonitis
3. medial ligament syndrome
4. popliteus sydrome.

Osteochondritis dissecans

This is more common in boys in the second decade. Pain with activity and clicking or giving are presenting symptoms. Clinically there is a mild effusion, usually with quadriceps wasting and tenderness over the site of the lesion (medial femoral condyle). Locking occurs if the fragment separates, with a loose body usually felt in the suprapatellar pouch. X-rays are usually diagnostic and tunnel views identify the intra-articular pathology in most cases. MRI will often confirm the diagnosis. An undisplaced fragment in the younger child is treated conservatively with rest. Loose fragments are replaced and fixed if possible or excised in the chronic case.

Osgood–Schlatter disease

This is a traction apophysitis of the tibial tuberosity, is seen in children 10–14 years, and is associated with overuse. There is pain with or without enlargement of the tibial tuberosity. X-ray usually shows characteristic fragmentation of the tuberosity. The symptoms usually settle with rest. Surgical excision of the fragments is rarely necessary in chronic disease.

Sindig–Larsen–Johansson syndrome

This is analogous to Osgood–Schlatter disease, but occurring at the distal pole of the patella.

Chondromalacia patellae

This is a pathological and descriptive term for softening of the patellar femoral articular cartilage and this diagnosis can only be made at arthroscopy or with histopathological examination. It is associated with anterior knee pain syndrome and with patellar instability and maltracking and is a feature of early degenerative patellar-femoral disease.

Bipartite patella

This normal variant is usually seen as a lucent line at the superolateral corner of the patella and can be mistaken for a fracture. It occurs when the ossification centres of the patella fail to fuse. Surgery is rarely required. This condition is often bilateral and an X-ray can be taken of both knees in order to differentiate between a developmental bipartite patellar and an acute fracture.

Plica syndrome

This is often diagnosed but is rarely a specific cause of knee pain. It is caused by failure of the breakdown of the embryonic synovial shelves which normally occurs by the fourth intrauterine month. Medial plica is most often implicated and the diagnosis is suspected by palpating a thickened band which may click or snap over the medial femoral condyle. A steroid injection should be tried, followed by arthroscopic division if this fails.

Septic arthritis and osteomyelitis

This is a relatively common disorder with infection, usually blood-borne, from the upper respiratory tract. The patient presents with severe pain and a tense effusion. The slightest movement causes agony and the patient is usually clearly unwell. Appropriate antibiotics should be commenced immediately and arthroscopic washout instigated as an emergency. The differential diagnosis includes other inflammatory pathologies, including non-specific synovitis and Still's disease.

Acute haematogenous osteomyelitis commonly affects the proximal tibial or distal femoral metaphyses. The patient is usually unwell with local tenderness and a high WBC and inflammatory markers (CRP and ESR).

Popliteal cysts and swellings (Baker's cyst)

This is a common finding which can occur at any age. Most cysts communicate with the knee joint and the semimembranosus bursa on the medial side of the knee is most often implicated. There is swelling with or without pain at the back of the knee, which is usually more prominent when the knee is extended. There may be restricted flexion. In children there is often no other abnormality but in the older patient, intra-articular pathology such as osteoarthritis is the norm. Differential diagnosis includes popliteal artery aneurysms and tumours. MRI is the investigation of choice if there is concern with the diagnosis. In children, most regress with time. In the adult, treatment should be directed at the underlying cause. Surgical excision is rarely required as the recurrence rate is high.

Synovial pathology

Recurrent effusions of spontaneous onset, with or without pain, can occur. Patients present with diffuse swelling and thickening, mainly felt above the patella, usually with quadriceps wasting and a mild flexion deformity.

Non-specific synovitis

This is a relatively common problem, of spontaneous onset, which occurs mainly in early adulthood. Patients may relate this to recent non-specific illness. Inflammatory blood screen is routine. It may settle with rest but a steroid injection may be required. Recurrent symptoms which fail with conservative treatment require arthroscopic synovectomy and synoid biopsy where histology shows non-specific features. Occasionally the condition may progress to an inflammatory picture such as rheumatoid arthritis. Surgery is usually curative.

Pigmented villonodular synovitis (PVNS)

This condition occurs most commonly in young adults who complain of pain and swelling and the knee is the most commonly involved joint. PVNS may involve the whole joint (diffuse) or present as a local intra-articular swelling (focal) disease. Clinical examination may reveal little apart from diffuse swelling and joint line pain. MRI examination gives a characteristic appearance and defines the extent of the disease. Arthroscopic synovial biopsy will confirm the diagnosis and arthroscopic synovectomy is the treatment of choice. With recurrent disease, open synovectomy and external beam radiotherapy and later joint replacement are occasionally indicated.

Synovial osteochrondromatosis

This is an uncommon metaplastic condition that most commonly affects the knee. Plain radiographs usually show multiple small loose bodies within and around the joint. These bodies are cartilage nodules which undergo calcification and ossification and become detached to form loose bodies within the joint. Clinical examination usually confirms synovial thickening and palpable loose bodies. Arthroscopic synovectomy and loose body removal is usually successful at alleviating the majority of the symptoms.

Table 7.3   Indications for knee replacement surgery

Pain	This is the main indication for surgery. Pain that occurs at rest and at night, which is refractory to analgesia and worse with movement or on weight bearing, is a strong indication for TKR
Activities of daily living	If the restricted movement and pain caused by the arthritis is significantly affecting the ability to walk, dress, wash, etc., then this is a relative indication for knee replacement
Instability	Lack of confidence with the knee, with recurrent giving way and locking and swelling of the joint is an indication for TKR
Age	Because joint replacements have limited survival (95% at 10 years), surgery under the age of 50 has to be considered carefully or alternative surgery such as high tibial osteotomy has to be considered

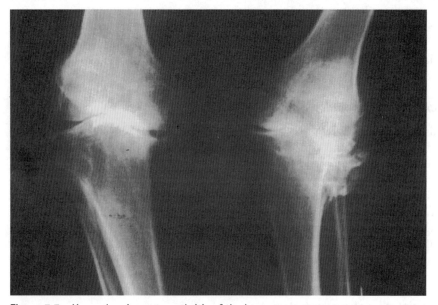

Figure 7.7   X-ray showing osteoarthritis of the knee

IMAGING

1. Routine X-rays in the young adult and soft tissue injuries are often normal.
2. Standard views should be weight bearing. The series should include AP, lateral, and skyline views of the patella if instability is suspected.

Table 7.4   Indications of problems with a knee replacement

Pain	Any significant and sustained increase in pain around a joint replacement should be investigated. If in doubt, refer. Some patients have a persistent ache in the lower limb, even with an otherwise successful joint replacement
Loss of movement	Artificial joints are often stiff but a sudden loss of movement should be investigated with a radiograph
Fracture	Fractures can occur around artificial joints, particularly if the implant is loose. They usually present acutely with severe pain, deformity and loss of function. Emergency referral is indicated
Loosening	Aseptic loosening of joint replacements occurs in about 5% of cases at 10 years. It will usually present with gradual onset of pain and should be investigated with an X-ray. If loosening is present then refer
Infection	Deep infection is rare after joint replacements (<3%). It will usually present with pain. Sometimes local signs are present. Rarely the patient may be systemically unwell, and emergency referral is indicated in these situations *Do not* treat with antibiotics and refer immediately if there is a high suspicion of deep infection so there is a greater chance of identifying the causative organism with knee aspiration
DVT and pulmonary embolus	DVT is common after lower limb joint replacement. Isolated calf vein thromboses can be treated conservatively but thrombi extending above the knee are best treated with anticoagulants (subcutaneous heparin and 6 months of warfarin). Deaths from pulmonary emboli are rare (<1%)

3. Supplementary views include intracondylar if a loose body is suspected, and a true lateral with the knee flexed at 30 degrees to assess for dysplasia in instability. Stress films should be included where significant ligamentous injury is suspected and oblique views with tibial plateau fractures.

Magnetic resonance imaging (MRI)

1. This is now an invaluable tool in assessing soft tissue injuries of the knee. It is sensitive and specific for meniscal and ligamentous injuries.
2. No ionizing radiation is utilized.
3. It is best for assessing soft tissue structures and intraosseous disease, including osteomyelitis, and tumours.

Computed tomography (CT)

1. This allows cross-section evaluation and is useful in assessing fractures of the knee.
2. Assessing bone-forming tumours.

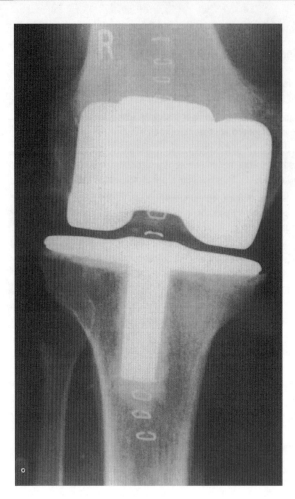

Figure 7.8   X-ray of total knee replacement

Nuclear medicine

1. This is best for evaluating the whole skeleton for multifocal disease.
2. A bone scan is useful in identifying stress fractures and RSD following knee injury.

Chapter 8

Foot and ankle

Paul H. Cooke

- Many foot problems can be treated by restoring anatomical alignment.
- Collapse of the medial arch is a common cause of hindfoot and midfoot pain.
- Calcaneal spurs are rarely of clinical significance.
- Forefoot surgery is a major procedure – recovery may take up to 6 months.
- Steroids should not be injected into the Achilles tendon.

PRESENTING SYMPTOMS

The adult foot and ankle make a complex structure, with joints allowing flexion and extension at the ankle, inversion and eversion at the subtalar joint, rotation at the mid-tarsal region, and fine movements of the toes. The interaction of the joints means that problems in different parts of the feet are frequently functionally and causally related. This, coupled with a complex language used to describe foot problems, has led to a mystique that problems of the foot must be dealt with by a specialist of one sort or another.

In truth, many problems can be solved simply if certain principles are followed. The principles are based on the observation that the 'normal' healthy foot functions well in practice, and that many foot problems can be treated by restoring anatomical alignment.

Corns, callosities and other such painful lesions only occur due to abnormal pressure from within or outside the foot.

COMMON FOOT AND ANKLE CONDITIONS

Hindfoot and midfoot pain

The common cause of pain in the hindfoot and midfoot is valgus hindfoot with collapse of the medial arch, which occurs in middle age and beyond. It is much commoner in women. The conditions are related, and one leads to the other if untreated. Both occur secondary to progressive weakness of the calf muscles.

Table 8.1   Common causes of foot and ankle pain in different age groups

Age group	Cause		
	Intra–articular	Periarticular	Referred
Childhood (2–10 years)	Club foot Congenital midfoot and forefoot deformities Septic arthritis	Osteomyelitis	
Adolescence (10–18 years)	Arch disorders (pes cavus, pes planus)	Osteomyelitis Tumours	
Early adulthood (18–30 years)	Metatarsalgia Hallux valgus Hallux rigidus Osteochondritis Accessory ossicles	Achilles tendonitis Achilles tendon rupture Fasciitis	Lumbar spine Knee
Adulthood (30–50 years)	Osteoarthritis Inflammatory arthritis Gout Metatarsalgia Hallux valgus Hallux rigidus Osteochondritis Accessory ossicles	Ischaemic foot pain Diabetes Bursitis Tendonitis Plantar fasciitis Corns	Lumbar spine Knee
Old age (>50 years)	Osteoarthritis Inflammatory arthritis Gout Metatarsalgia Hallux valgus Hallux rigidus	Ischaemic foot pain Diabetes Bursitis Tendonitis Plantar fasciitis Corns	Lumbar spine Knee

The patient describes foot pain which increases on walking, and which may restrict walking distance.

Assessment should be made of the position and angulations of the hindfoot and midfoot when standing. The patient is observed from behind, and a visual line dropped vertically from the centre of the knee joint. This should pass through the centre of the ankle joint (and Achilles tendon) and to the centre of the heel. Commonly, when the hindfoot is painful, the ankle/subtalar joint is in valgus, so the imaginary line passes medial to the ankle joint. If this deformity is observed, test to see whether this can be corrected passively with the patient sitting.

Next the patient should turn round to face the examiner, and the arch of the foot should be observed. The patient should be asked whether the arch has 'dropped' compared with their normal stance. The arch should be observed with the heels on the ground, and then on standing on tiptoes. This assesses the mobility of the arch.

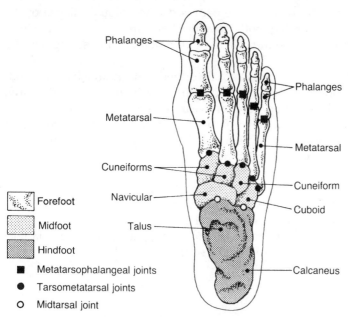

Figure 8.1   Bone joints and regions of the foot

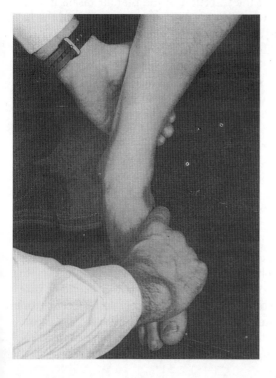

Figure 8.2   Testing for ankle instability

Treatment depends on whether the pain is due to valgus collapse of the hindfoot, collapse of the arch or both. The objective of treatment is to position the foot beneath the leg, with the sole flat to the floor, and to strengthen the weak muscles.

Method 1   If the subtalar joint is not deformed, but the arch has dropped, supply an arch support. Many shoes contain an arch support. Medial arch supports can be easily obtained from footwear or surgical appliance shops.

Method 2   If the subtalar joint is valgus, then the heel needs supporting in a vertical position. If the deformity is minor then it may again be corrected by a medial arch support which will force the heel into line. For more severe deformities the heel must also be directly supported. This may be achieved by supplying custom-made splints (extended heel cups – extended forwards to include an arch support), or by wearing running training shoes, as these incorporate a firm heel counter and a firm medial arch support.

Whichever of these methods is adopted, the patient must be taught foot and calf exercises, or the relief and support from the orthoses will be short-lived.

Painful heel

Painful heel, plantar fasciitis, or policeman's heel most commonly occurs in men in their fifties or sixties. It is characterized by pain beneath the heel worse on standing. The site of the pain can often be pinpointed exactly. The pain probably reflects excess tension at the insertion of the plantar fascia into the calcaneum. This is secondary to weakness of the intrinsic muscles of the calf and foot, allowing the arch to sag and creating tightening in the plantar fascia.

On examination no abnormality can be detected other than a severely painful area beneath the heel. Radiographs should generally be avoided unless there are atypical features such as pain at night. X-ray will often show a calcaneal spur, but only because it is such a common finding anyway. Patients may become fixated on this spur despite its being of no clinical significance.

Treatment of mild cases comprises anti-inflammatory medication, physiotherapy with foot and calf exercises and local ultrasound. On occasions improvement in symptoms may be obtained by wearing silicone or foam rubber heel pads. In more severe cases these can be trimmed centrally to give them the appearance of a horseshoe. By this means the weight is carried completely away from the tender area.

Some cases are severe and do not respond to these treatments. For these patients, treatment is by injection of the painful area with local anaesthetic and steroid. This is effective but is itself painful. Few patients will wish to have the injection repeated and for this reason a long-acting depot steroid should be used.

The natural history of this condition is that it rarely lasts longer than 18 months or 2 years, provided surgical treatment is not undertaken. The outcome of surgical treatment is poor. Release of the plantar fascia can lead to a chronically painful flat foot, lasting far beyond 2 years. For this reason referral is usually only worthwhile for provision of orthoses, or for further injection to be administered under anaesthetic.

Forefoot problems

Bunions

Bunions are a common condition in Caucasians. They may be transmitted in families by autosomal dominant inheritance with variable penetrance. Patients present with symptoms relating to rubbing of the bunion on shoes or with concern about the natural history and progression of bunions, wanting treatment before they 'get as bad as granny's'.

Patients with bunions should be examined as described above for hindfoot and midfoot pain. Both heel valgus and flat foot make bunions worse and may indeed cause them. In patients with a flat foot or valgus heel, correction of the medial arch will often correct the hallux valgus, reduce the width of the forefoot and ease the pain from the bunion.

To demonstrate whether an arch support would be effective the patient is made to stand with a small roll of foam beneath the medial arch of the foot. Alternatively the examiner's fingers can be held in the same place supporting the medial arch. The degree of correctability can thus be demonstrated. If correction is obtained then a medial arch support should help. If there is no correction, and symptoms are severe enough to warrant surgical treatment, then the patient should be referred for a specialist opinion. Patients should be aware that forefoot surgery is a major, and on occasions painful, undertaking. Most operations require plaster or splintage for about 8 weeks, then a further

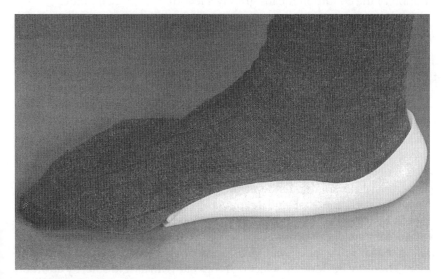

Figure 8.3   Heel cup for valgus heel deformity

Table 8.2   Normal range of movement: forefoot

| Inversion | 0–35 degrees |
| Eversion | 0–15 degrees |

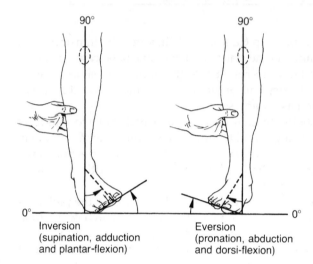

90°   90°

Inversion   Eversion
(supination, adduction   (pronation, abduction
and plantar-flexion)   and dorsi-flexion)

0°   0°

Figure 8.4   (a) Inversion (supination, adduction and plantarflexion); (b) eversion (pronation, abduction and dorsiflexion)

8 weeks until a shoe can be worn for a whole day. It is often 6 months or more before the foot has recovered to the preoperative level of function.

Patients should not be referred because of worries about future progression of mild bunions. Progression is extremely variable, so surgery on minor bunions as a preventative manoeuvre would be inappropriate. In any case, the variable penetration of the condition means granny's feet may be no real guide.

Hallux rigidus

Hallux rigidus is a common painful condition of degenerative arthritis of the first metatarsophalangeal (MTP) joint, commonly occurring in the dominant foot of sports-orientated young men in their twenties and early thirties. It causes pain, particularly on kneeling with the toe tucked beneath the foot, and also when crouching or running.

The diagnosis can be confirmed by palpation of the first MTP joint. A ridge of osteophyte will be felt circumferentially. Unlike the osteophyte palpable in hallux valgus (the bunion), the osteophyte of hallux rigidus can be felt on the dorsum and dorsolateral side of the joint. The joint is always tender on palpation between the first and second toes. Similarly, dorsiflexion of the great toe is restricted and painful.

Symptomatic relief can be obtained by advising the patient to keep their toe straight when kneeling (and not to tuck it beneath the foot), or by stiffening the footwear. This may be done by selecting footwear with a rigid sole, by addition of a stiffening bar to the sole of the shoe or by insertion of a rigid insole.

If the patient develops rest and night pain or pain which interferes with work, then surgical referral is advised. Surgery is usually similar to bunion surgery, and the same recovery period applies. In some centres arthroscopic surgery for minor cases is now becoming popular.

Metatarsalgia

Metatarsalgia is a condition in which pain is felt beneath the metatarsal heads. It may occur beneath a single metatarsal or beneath two or more metatarsals. Commonly it occurs in patients who have a high arch (a cavus foot). The patient usually describes a feeling as though they are 'walking on a pebble'. The diagnosis is made from the history. Examination of the foot may reveal a high arch and in more severe cases, corns or calluses beneath the metatarsal heads. In severe cases and those associated with generalized arthropathies, dislocation of the MTP joints may occur.

Treatment is directed to relief of pain. In many patients, good relief can be obtained by trimming the calluses. If the outcome from such chiropody is maintained, particularly in elderly or unfit patients, no further measures may be required. Additional help may be obtained by the use of metatarsal pads. These come in two forms. The first is a pad with adhesive backing which is inserted into the shoe. The second is a pad on an elastic strap which is held beneath the foot by passing the elastic strapping around the forefoot. Such pads are often sold with inadequate instructions, and it is important to advise the patient that the pad must be worn behind the area of pain, thus transferring the weight through the pad into the metatarsal neck. If, as commonly happens, it is worn beneath the corn or tender area then it will simply increase the problem.

The patient should be referred if they do not respond to local measures or pads.

Morton's neuroma

A small number of patients who have symptoms similar to metatarsalgia complain of a severe lancinating pain radiating down into the cleft between two toes. It is accompanied by numbness of the adjoining skin of the two toes. This is caused by a benign inflammatory neuroma of the interdigital nerve (a Morton's neuroma).

This is diagnosed by compression of the metatarsals causing pain. Pain can also be induced by pressure on the sole of the foot in the interdigital area.

Neuromas can be treated by injection with local anaesthetic and steroid. The neuroma is palpated from the sole of the foot and the injection is made through the dorsum of the foot on to the identified point. The neuroma lies deep to the skin on the sole of the foot, so the injection needs to be deep into the foot. Ultrasound examination will confirm or exclude a neuroma, and an accurate injection can be performed at the same time. The radiologist can see the neuroma at the time of injection and can therefore inject accurately and avoid painful intraneural injection.

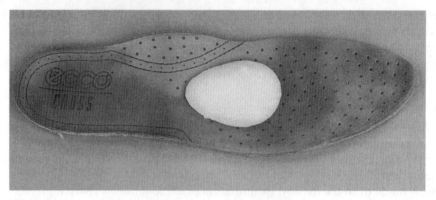

Figure 8.5   Insole with metatarsal dome

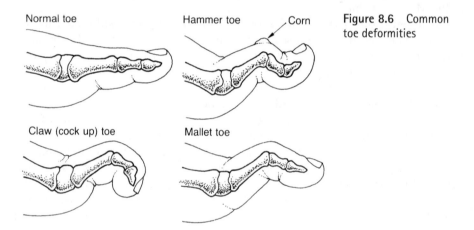

Figure 8.6   Common toe deformities

If the pain fails to respond, or there is later remission, referral for a surgical opinion is required.

Toe deformities

Deformities of the lesser toes may be categorized and described as follows (Figure 8.6):

1. curly toes – toes which curl into flexion but which are passively correctable
2. claw toes – curly toes which are uncorrectable
3. hammer toes – toes in which there is flexion of the proximal interphalangeal joint and extension of the distal interphalangeal joint
4. mallet toes – where there is flexion of the distal interphalangeal joint only.

Deformities of the toes are only important when they rub on the footwear. Hammer toes frequently develop corns on the dorsum of the proximal

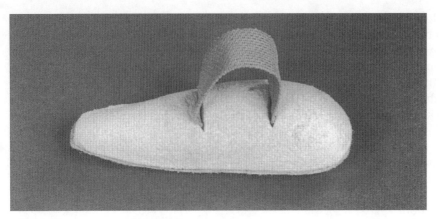

Figure 8.7   Hammer toe splint

Figure 8.8   Banana splint for curly toes

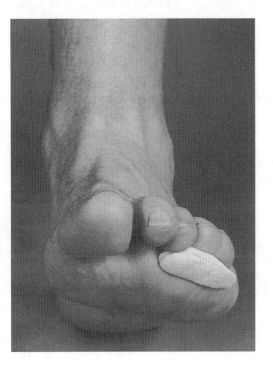

interphalangeal joint. Claw toes have callosities and corns over the dorsum of the proximal interphalangeal joint or beneath the tip of the toe (where the soft skin of the tip of the toe is directed into the sole of the shoe). Mallet toes have corns on the tip of the toe.

Treatment is aimed at relieving pain, by protecting the painful area or by surgery. Local chiropody may provide temporary relief when a hard corn rubs, but often it is the better long-term option to correct the toes surgically unless the patient is very frail. When palliation alone is appropriate, or when problems arise only with certain footwear (e.g. walking boots), then corn pads may protect the skin. Modern silicone tubes and pads are more effective than foam pads which tend to harden when compressed.

It may be appropriate to buy shoes with a high toe cap to prevent rubbing of the dorsum of the toe on the shoe, and/or to use a soft 'banana' splint (which tucks beneath curly or clawed toes), to lift the tips of the toes from the sole of the shoe.

In fit patients with substantial symptoms, referral for surgery is indicated to obviate long-term conservative treatment. Because the risk of infection in the toes is high, elderly patients who have joint replacements elsewhere in the body should also be referred, as surgery may prevent the chance of secondary infection.

Traditional fusion/correction of the toes requires a pin in the toes for 8 weeks. This needs to be removed later. More recently, techniques avoiding the use of pins have been developed and these reduce the high infection rate of pins and speed up recovery.

Ingrown toenails

Ingrown toenails are almost limited to the great toenail. They are predisposed to by flattening of the arch (when the great toe is rolled over), by pressure from ill-fitting shoes or by trauma. They often present with acute infection with chronic granulation.

It is important to identify predisposing events such as a new pair of ill-fitting shoes or poor pedicure, and the foot should be examined for predisposing hindfoot or midfoot deformities. The nail should be observed end-on to assess the curvature of the edge of the nail. Nails which substantially curl down at the edges are unlikely to respond to local treatment.

Local measures such as curettage of the nail or simple wedge resection may be tried with a reasonable prospect of success if a predisposing factor has been identified and can be avoided in the future. Simple removal is indicated for a single episode of ingrown toenail in adolescence or adulthood, but there is no place for undertaking recurrent removals of the nail.

If recurrences of ingrowing toenail occur, then removal with nail bed ablation should be performed. The choice as to whether this should be wedge resections or complete resections should be discussed with the patient. The risk of recurrence is greater with wedge resections although the cosmetic result is better.

Achilles tendon problems

Two conditions particularly affect the Achilles tendon, namely Achilles tendonitis and Achilles tendon rupture. It is believed that both are ruptures of fibres of the Achilles tendon. In Achilles tendonitis, just one or two fibres rupture at a time, causing severe pain and an inflammatory response.

Achilles tendonitis

The patient with Achilles tendonitis may be any age. It often arises after excessive use. Thus it may occur in younger people training for marathons or road running but equally it may occur in the elderly. The patient describes severe pain around the Achilles tendon which often increases on standing on tiptoes. There is usually a diffuse swelling around the tendon and it is always locally tender.

It is important to differentiate this from tendon rupture. This can be done by the squeeze or Thompson's test. The patient lies face down on the couch with their feet hanging over the end of the couch. If the normal calf is squeezed firmly then the foot will plantarflex. With a ruptured tendon, squeezing the calf will lead to at most a tiny flicker of movement. Although there are other tests for Achilles tendon rupture, they are less reliable and this is the definitive test.

Having excluded tendon rupture, the patient should be treated by reducing their level of activities and with anti-inflammatory medication. Many patients find it more comfortable to raise the heel slightly. Often a different pair of shoes with a higher heel is more comfortable. Fashion victims with only flat heeled shoes may find a cushioned heel insole such as that used for policeman's heel is effective. If these measures fail, then a period of 4 weeks in plaster of paris almost always cures the problem.

Steroids should not be injected into the Achilles tendon, as this may precipitate tendon rupture (which is actually rare without steroid injections).

Referral to a specialist is usually unnecessary unless this is the only way to gain access to a plaster of paris.

On occasions Achilles tendonitis is accompanied by a feeling of nodules in the tendon. These reflect small ruptures which have healed and calcified. They are extremely unlikely to be cancerous as tumours of the Achilles tendon are

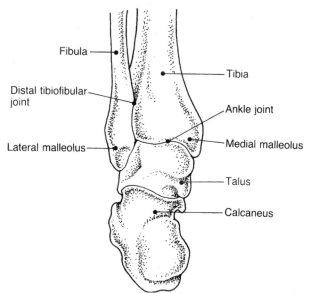

Fibula

Tibia

Distal tibiofibular joint

Ankle joint

Lateral malleolus

Medial malleolus

Talus

Calcaneus

Figure 8.9   The bones of the ankle

Table 8.3 Normal range of movement: ankle

Plantarflexion	0–50 degrees
Dorsiflexion	0–20 degrees

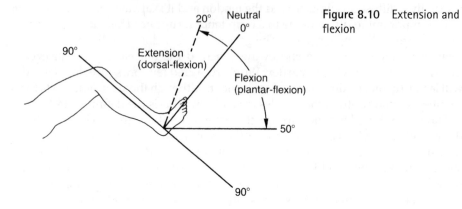

Figure 8.10 Extension and flexion

rare, making referral unnecessary. The diagnosis can be excluded unless there has been rapid growth of a lump beyond 2 cm.

Achilles tendon rupture

Achilles tendon rupture happens much more commonly in men, usually around their forties. However, it can affect a wide range of people. The commonest history is the feeling of a snap or being struck behind the heel, often while playing badminton or squash. Players may think their opponent has hit them with their racquet and have been known to retaliate. Rupture can also follow other accidents. The commonest of these is missing a step on a ladder or the rung breaking. The common feature of all these activities is forced sudden dorsiflexion of the foot.

The back of the heel is always tender and swollen. Thompson's test (as described above and also sometimes known as Simmond's test) is always positive, and this should always be performed. Although surgeons differ as to whether they should treat tendon ruptures conservatively or surgically, all would agree that they must be treated promptly and actively. Thus, any patient with an Achilles tendon rupture should be referred to hospital within 24 hours or so.

The results of surgical treatment are heavily affected by the degree of the swelling and the state of the soft tissues, and for this reason it is important to elevate the leg as much as possible and if possible pack it with cold compresses or ice packs to reduce soft tissue damage while awaiting transfer. A bag of frozen peas from the freezer wrapped in a towel and applied for 10 minutes is a classical solution, though other frozen vegetables may suffice.

Whether surgery is undertaken or not, the patient will need to be in plaster for 8–12 weeks after an Achilles tendon rupture.

In some series, up to half of all Achilles tendon ruptures have been missed. The possibility of a delayed presentation should be considered in any patient who has sprained their ankle and continues to limp. Again, a Thompson's test will be positive. However, there is a pitfall for the unwary. If the tendon itself is examined more than 3 months after the rupture then it will feel intact. When a Thompson's test is performed, it may be assumed that the Achilles tendon had not ruptured. In fact, what will have happened is that the tendon has ruptured and then healed in its lengthened state. Squeezing the calf will still lead to a negative result. The patient will be disabled with a permanent limp unless surgery is undertaken.

The decision as to whether to operate on a missed rupture is increasingly difficult as time passes from rupture to presentation. However, these patients warrant urgent referral to an orthopaedic surgeon.

Chapter 9

Children

Michael K. D. Benson

- A typical finding of bone/joint sepsis is pseudoparalysis.
- Back pain associated with scoliosis indicates serious pathology in children.
- Clicky hips rarely matter, hip instability does.
- Fifty per cent of limping children with knee pain will have hip pathology.
- Nocturnal limb pains in children are common, often transitory, and in the absence of clinical findings require reassurance.

PRESENTING SYMPTOMS

It is a trite but true comment that children are not just little adults. A range of conditions affects children uniquely and growth modifies the child's response to deformity, infection and injury.

Children are often better historians than their parents: when possible listen to the child's account of the problem and not the parent's interpretation.

Children may feel threatened by unfamiliar surroundings. While bright lights and an examination couch help the doctor, the child is almost always happier on his or her mother's lap. It is sensible always to leave the unpleasant part of an examination until the end: abduct the child's hips at the end of the examination, not at the beginning.

Children both recover from and deteriorate quickly with illness. If, for example, bone or joint sepsis is suspected, it is always wise to re-examine a child a few hours later when the situation has clarified.

ORTHOPAEDIC PROBLEMS IN CHILDREN OF ANY AGE

Infection

Bone and joint infections are serious at any age and need urgent hospital admission. If the diagnosis is suspected the child should always be referred as an emergency. It is a mistake to treat blindly with antibiotics. Blind antibiotic treatment may obscure the causative organism and make the correct selection of antibiotics almost impossible.

In the neonate and young infant the diagnosis of infection may be difficult. Fever is not invariably present but the child is unhappy and listless. A typical finding is pseudoparalysis: the child does not voluntarily move the affected joint. In the case, for example, of shoulder sepsis, Erb's palsy may mistakenly be diagnosed. In a superficial joint or bone of an older child the diagnosis is usually obvious because of local swelling and tenderness. In a deeply placed joint, even in the older child, restriction of joint movement may be the only pointer to the diagnosis. Bone and joint infection is almost always blood borne but often the primary focus of infection cannot be identified.

Tumours

Benign bone tumours are not rare in childhood. They almost never cause symptoms until they present with a pathological fracture following a minor injury. Some benign tumours, like hereditary multiple exostoses, are familial.

Malignant bone and soft tissue tumours are rare in infancy and childhood, but become slightly more common in adolescence. All types of bone tumour are most common about the knee where most skeletal growth occurs. Bone tumours should be suspected if pain is present both at night and in the day and if there is local bone thickening and tenderness. Clearly it would be inappropriate for every child with knee-ache to be X-rayed, but aching unrelated to exercise or activity which causes night discomfort should trigger alarm bells.

Scoliosis

Congenital scoliosis may be apparent at birth. It is associated with abnormalities of individual vertebrae, so that they are either partially conjoined or absent. Angular deformity may be demonstrable but rotation is often not prominent. Such vertebral anomalies may be associated with spina bifida.

It is sensible during any routine developmental check on a child to examine the spine but routine school screening for scoliosis, the so-called 'schooliosis', is no longer practised. The problem is that many children have mild spinal asymmetry, requiring no treatment, and spinal surgeons were overwhelmed by demand when all such children were referred to them. If any spinal curve is detected, provided it is trivial it does not need referral. It is, however, essential that the child be observed over time by the general practitioner and if there is any hint of progression then referral becomes appropriate. Particular care should be taken in adolescence when rapid curvature may develop.

Back pain is an unusual symptom in children and if it is associated with scoliosis there is likely to be a significant underlying spinal problem. The combination of pain and scoliosis demands specialist referral as spinal infection, tumour or intrathecal abnormality may underlie this combination of complaints.

Rickets and metabolic bone disease

Dietary rickets is extremely rare in the UK. Familial vitamin D-resistant rickets is less rare and, unlike children with dietary rickets, those with hypophosphataemic rickets are bright and cheerful and have no proximal muscle weakness. Pronounced deformity in the weight-bearing lower limbs is common, with anterolateral femoral bowing and internal torsion, along with bowing of the tibia, the most common deformities. The bony deformities are symmetrical and progressive unless halted by diagnosis and appropriate treatment. Similar bone deformities may occur in children with renal impairment.

Any child of abnormal stature, whether too tall or too small or with limb/trunk length disproportion, should be referred to a growth expert, as there are a vast number of rare skeletal dysplasias with additional variants being regularly described.

AGE-RELATED PROBLEMS

Infancy

Congenital anomalies

Most congenital orthopaedic problems are easily seen. Extra digits, syndactyly and missing parts are obvious. A deep dimple or pit may reflect an underlying bony deficit. Deep dimples in the buttocks, for example, may suggest an absent sacrum. Deformities at the hip and spine may be more difficult to detect. The spine is most easily checked with the child held prone and flopping down on the examiner's hand. It is easy to check for scoliosis. It is also easy to palpate the spine, feeling for absent spinous processes, suggesting an underlying spina bifida. Skin blemishes such as patches of pigmentation or hairy tufts should alert the examiner to the possibility of an underlying spinal and neurological defect. It is wise to check for postanal pits and dimples: if these are not blind ending, neurosurgical advice should be sought. It is important to remember that occult spinal abnormalities in infancy may not be associated with a neurological deficit. However, if abnormal cord tethering is present, neurological symptoms and signs may develop with growth.

It is very important to remember that if a child has one congenital anomaly others are likely.

Children are amazingly malleable after birth and postural deformity is common. The prone-lying child tends to develop hooked forefeet or metatarsus adductus. The side-lying child readily develops an eccentric skull shape, a postural scoliosis and asymmetry in hip abduction. Parents should be encouraged to alternate the sleeping position of their children. Children should keep either on their backs or on alternate sides until old enough to turn themselves.

The hips

In 1969 a circular to all doctors advised that every infant's hips should be carefully examined by the manoeuvres described by Ortolani and Barlow. It was believed that this would prevent the late presentation of all children with congenital hip dislocation. These recommendations are under review but it is currently advised that all children should have their hips examined at birth and before discharge from hospital. They should subsequently be examined at 6–8 weeks, 6–8 months and thereafter at 18–24 months. New screening criteria will shortly be in use: babies should have their hips examined at birth and at the 6-week check. All examinations will have to be performed by a team fully trained in the techniques of management.

It is, however, important that all clinicians who deal with children are competent in hip examination techniques. As background it is worth noting that 2% of all children have hips which are demonstrably unstable at birth. Fortunately the great majority of these resolve with no treatment. If no screening is performed, however, 1–2 per 1000 are left with displaced hips and a further 1–2 present in later life with premature arthritis as a consequence of hip dysplasia. The fashionable term for describing the range of hip instability and dysplasia is now 'developmental dysplasia of the hip' (DDH). The important point to remember when examining the child's hip is that one is testing the relationship between the femoral head and the acetabulum. The hip is either in joint and stable, in joint but displaceable, out of joint but reducible or out of joint and irreducible. The most common error is to feel for a click. Clicks rarely matter, instability does!

If hip instability is not recognizable at birth, within a few weeks fixed displacement of the hip joint occurs and the cardinal signs change. The child's leg may be slightly short, externally rotated and have asymmetrical thigh creases (however, one in three normal children has asymmetrical thigh creases). If the hip is displaced the critical clinical sign is restriction of abduction when the hip is flexed.

If ever there is doubt about a child's hip it is wise to refer for specialist examination. In the child over the age of 4 months it would be entirely reasonable to request an X-ray evaluation and to refer to a specialist only if the X-ray is abnormal.

It is of course worth remembering the risk factors for hip instability. These include a positive family history, oligohydramnios, a breech presentation or a deformity of the foot.

The knees and feet

Knee deformities are rare at birth. Hyperextended or dislocated knees may be seen in association with neurological abnormalities or an extended breech.

By contrast foot deformities are common. The most frequent is talipes calcaneovalgus (talipes = talus + pes = ankle + foot). The calcaneovalgus foot is directed upwards and outwards and needs nothing other than simple stretching. Almost all resolve within a matter of a few weeks. As noted before, it may be associated with hip instability.

Talipes equinovarus or club foot occurs in 2 per 1000 children and is sometimes familial. It is increasingly spotted antenatally by ultrasound. Club feet

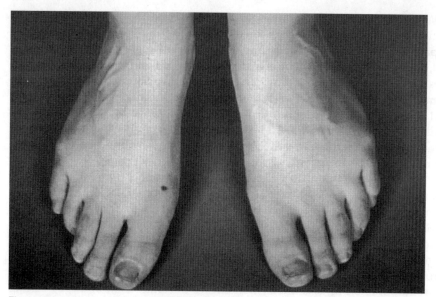

Figure 9.1   Curly fourth toes which very rarely require treatment

need specialist treatment by serial stretching, strapping, plaster or physio-therapy and many will need surgery in the first few months of life. It is import-ant to note that a true structural club foot will always be smaller than its counterpart and that calf wasting is an integral part of the problem.

Minor toe deformities are common: the second toe often appears high rid-ing but needs no treatment. Curliness of the fourth and fifth toes is often familial and certainly needs no treatment in infancy. Provided the infant's foot is supple and flexible it is unlikely to be a problem. If it is stiff and inflexible, expert advice should be sought, as there may be underlying bony coalition or a neuromuscular deficit.

The toddler

Walking is a critical age of childhood development. Parents are concerned by late walking. Bottom-shuffling children frequently do not walk independently until over 18 months. Any child who has not walked by 2 years, however, needs specialist evaluation by a paediatrician to ensure there is no neuromuscular abnormality.

When children start walking many problems come to light. Parents may be concerned by bandiness, knock-knees, in-toeing, out-toeing or flat foot. It is important to remember there is a normal physiological development: most children are slightly bandy when they start to walk but they may appear to be slightly knock-kneed by the age of 2–3 years. This resolves slowly over the course of the next 4–5 years.

When assessing apparent angular deformity one should always look for symmetry. Asymmetrical knock-knee may, for example, be the consequence of partial growth arrest or injury and needs specialist referral. When symmetrical, provided the bones themselves appear straight and the angular deformities are slight, there is no indication for referral. In a bandy child it is sensible to measure the distance between the knees when the ankles are just touching and in the knock-kneed child to measure the distance between the medial malleoli when the knees are just touching. There is rarely a cause for concern if the gap between the knees in a bandy child is 5 cm or less and in a knock-kneed child if the ankle gap is 7 cm or less.

In-toeing is common and is associated with either femoral torsion or internal tibial torsion. Both seem to be more common in lax-jointed children. Femoral torsion is simply judged by lying the child on his or her back with the knee flexed over the end of the couch and the hips extended. The hip can then be rotated internally and externally by rotating the leg like the hand of a clock. In general, the range of internal and external rotation is similar. Frequently it is found that the range of internal rotation considerably exceeds that of external rotation. It is this asymmetry that allows the child to sit in the TV sitting position, to walk with the toes turned in and to run with legs flicking sideways. The great majority of children need no treatment as there is spontaneous improvement over the first 7–10 years.

Internal tibial torsion may be judged with the child in the same position by dorsiflexing the foot and by checking which position the foot faces with regard to the knee. The average child will have 20 degrees of external torsion but there is a wide range of normal. It is not uncommon to see children with 40–50 degrees of internal torsion at toddler age yet the vast majority of these improve by school age. It is actually surprisingly uncommon for children to trip themselves up by catching one foot behind the opposite leg.

The limping child

The child who limps must always be taken seriously. The limp may reflect anything from a minor ankle sprain to hip sepsis. Beware of the child who complains of knee pain: at least half of such children will have a hip problem rather than a knee problem. Careful detailed analysis will usually allow the site of the problem, if not the diagnosis, to be clarified. Failure to examine the hip in this situation can have major consequences for the child.

In the absence of trauma the hip is by far the most frequent source of the problem in the limping toddler. Differential diagnoses include hip dislocation, sepsis, the irritable hip and Perthes' disease (idiopathic avascular necrosis). The dislocated hip should be easy to diagnose by identifying leg shortness with restricted abduction but without pain. It may be difficult to distinguish between the other three diagnoses. If the child appears healthy it is entirely reasonable to wait a few hours and re-examine. If hip discomfort has increased, the child has become unwell and the range of hip movement has decreased, then urgent referral and admission is mandatory. Of all joints that may be affected by infection the hip is the most problematical. Infection may lead to the destruction of the femoral head by avascular necrosis within 48 hours unless surgical decompression is urgently undertaken.

In practice, by toddler age, the signs of an infected hip are usually clear. The child is febrile, unwell and unhappy and there will be little doubt that they need urgent admission. It can be very difficult, however, to distinguish between the irritable hip and Perthes' disease. Again if the child is healthy, observation for a few days is sensible, referring on a semi-urgent basis if hip movement does not improve steadily.

The irritable hip remains one of the enigmas of childhood. It is alternatively known as transient synovitis and the observation hip. A small joint effusion is demonstrable by ultrasound. Aspiration may relieve the symptoms when a tense effusion is present. Only occasionally does a radiologically normal irritable hip progress to Perthes' disease. Perthes' disease is equally enigmatic but may lead to considerable disability and needs specialist supervision.

The foot

The flat foot is physiologically normal in children under 3 years. Children need referral only if the flat footedness is associated with pain, stiffness or grossly uneven shoe wear.

The night pains of childhood

These puzzling pains may be very distressing for the child and family. Typically the 2–8-year-old child wakes at night complaining of pain in one or other limb. The dutiful parent reassures the distressed child, massages the child's leg and sometimes gives simple analgesics. Within 30 or 40 minutes the discomfort has resolved and the child falls asleep to wake refreshed and bright in the morning, unlike the parent. The symptoms fluctuate. Pain may occur on two to three nights in succession and then be absent for 2–3 weeks. There is almost never significant discomfort by day and the child does not limp. Often there is a family history. It is the variable nocturnal pattern of pain which allows the diagnosis to be made and the parents' instinctive management is almost invariably correct.

The older child and adolescent

As the child gets older trauma becomes increasingly important. It is rare for an infant or young child to fracture a bone. Indeed, a femoral or tibial fracture in infancy needs careful evaluation to ensure that abuse has not contributed to the injury. As the child becomes physically more adventurous fractures become more common. Boys fracture more often than girls. Stress fractures are rare before adolescence. As they grow older, children may develop discomfort where tendons insert into growing areas of bone or apophyses. Traction apophysitis at the heel (Sever's disease), at the knee (Osgood–Schlatter

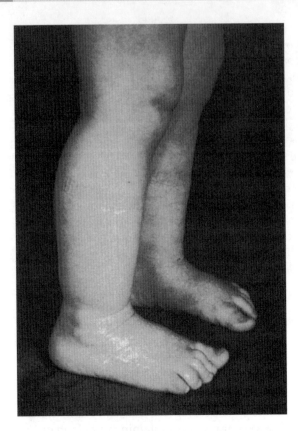

Figure 9.2   Infantile flat foot which rarely requires treatment

disease) or at the patella (Sinding–Larsen disease) are common in the 9–14-year age group. Meniscal injuries become more frequent at the same age. In the child who complains of clicking or locking at the knee under the age of 10, it is not uncommon to find a pathological discoid lateral meniscus, but in adolescents tearing of a normal meniscus is more likely. It is worth remembering that pain and swelling of the knee, ankle or elbow may occur with osteochondritis dissecans: a small fragment of bone adjacent to the joint surface becomes avascular and may separate with the overlying articular cartilage to create a loose body inside the joint.

Perthes' disease of the hip is rare after the age of 10 years. This is just as well as the prognosis deteriorates with age. Just as Perthes' disease fades in the diagnostic spectrum, so slipped upper femoral epiphysis appears. The child, often but not invariably overweight, complains of a limp and discomfort at the knee. Careful examination reveals that the leg is held in external rotation at the hip and is a little short. Movement at the hip is restricted. The usual delay between onset of symptoms and specialist referral is 6 months. This is sad, as the slipped upper femoral epiphysis, if diagnosed early, can be treated simply but if diagnosed later may cause considerable management problems and lead to premature arthritis. It should be high on the list of diagnostic possibilities and prompt X-ray and referral organized if it is suspected.

Chapter 10

Common orthopaedic injections
Jonathan Rees

Musculoskeletal injections of steroid and local anaesthetic can be diagnostic and therapeutic for certain orthopaedic pathologies. This chapter describes the methods of local injection for the treatment of some common conditions.* They can be performed by a primary care consultant often eliminating the need for orthopaedic referral.

Injection treatments for the following conditions are now described:

- impingement syndrome
- rotator cuff tears
- calcific tendonitis
- shoulder arthritis
- adhesive capsulitis (frozen shoulder)
- tennis elbow
- golfer's elbow
- arthritis of the thumb carpometacarpal joint
- De Quervain's tenosynovitis
- trigger finger or thumb
- carpal tunnel syndrome.

Note: for the following examples, aseptic technique must be followed; ml = millilitres and mg = milligrams. Avoid injecting subcutaneously – it is painful and is more likely to cause trophic skin changes.

UPPER LIMB: SHOULDER

 ### Posterior injection into the subacromial bursa

Indication

Impingement syndrome, rotator cuff tears and calcific tendonitis.

---

* Video clips of some of the techniques can be viewed at http://evolve.elsevier.com/Carr/orthopaedics/

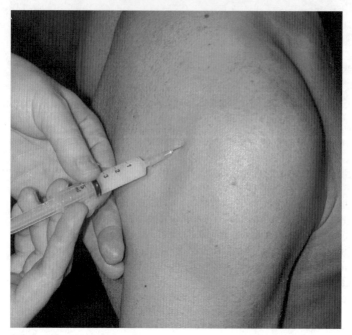

Figure 10.1   Posterior injection into the subacromial bursa

Technique

The posterior approach to the subacromial bursa is easier and generally safer. The entry point is 1 cm inferior and medial to the posterior corner of the acromion, or one finger-breadth down and one finger-breadth medially. Pass an 18-gauge needle up under the acromion to its full depth.

Use a combination of 2–5 ml of 1% lidocaine (lignocaine) mixed with **either**: 50 mg hydrocortisone acetate, **or** 20 mg triamcinolone, **or** 40 mg methylprednisolone.

Frequency

Every 4–6 weeks. If there is no benefit after two or three injections, then consider alternative treatment or referral.

Structure at risk

Injection directly into bone or periosteum is exquisitely painful and should be avoided. Also injecting under pressure into the tendon has a theoretical risk of causing tendon damage.

 Posterior injection into the glenohumeral joint

Indication

Arthritis or adhesive capsulitis (frozen shoulder).

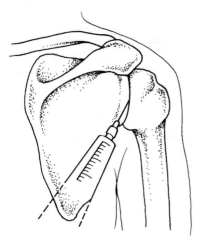

Figure 10.2   Injection of glenohumeral joint: posterior approach

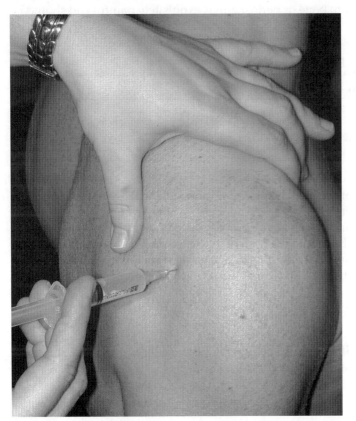

Figure 10.3   Posterior injection into the glenohumeral joint

Technique

The entry point is 1 cm inferior and medial to the posterior corner of the acromion, or one finger-breadth down and one finger-breadth medial. Put the index finger of your free hand on the corocoid process anteriorly and aim towards it up to the full depth of an 18-gauge needle. This will take you into the glenohumeral joint.

Use a combination of 2–5 ml of 1% lidocaine (lignocaine) mixed with **either**: 50 mg hydrocortisone acetate, **or** 20 mg triamcinolone, **or** 40 mg methyl-prednisolone.

Frequency

Every 4–6 weeks. If there is no benefit after two or three injections, then consider alternative treatment or referral.

Structures at risk

Injection directly into bone or periosteum is exquisitely painful and should be avoided.

UPPER LIMB: ELBOW

Medial injection at the elbow

Indication

Golfer's elbow (medial epicondylitis).

Technique

Palpate the point of the medial epicondyle and feel the fleshy substance of the flexor muscles anteriorly. The most tender area is often over the periosteum just anterior to the medial epicondyle. However, the pathology is in the muscle and you should aim to inject into the flesh of the flexor muscle to a depth of 1 cm.

Use a combination of 2 ml of 1% lidocaine (lignocaine) mixed with **either**: 10–25 mg hydrocortisone acetate, **or** 5–10 mg triamcinolone, **or** 10–20 mg methyl-prednisolone.

Frequency

Every 4–6 weeks. If there is no benefit after two or three injections, then consider alternative treatment or referral.

Structures at risk

Injection directly into bone or periosteum is exquisitely painful and should be avoided. Also, injecting under pressure into the tendon has a theoretical risk of causing tendon damage.

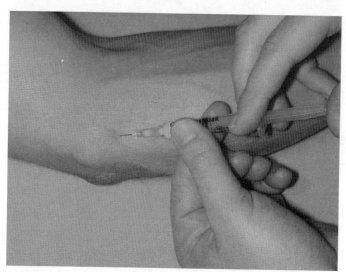

Figure 10.4   Injection for golfer's elbow (medial epicondylitis)

Try to avoid injecting subcutaneously over the medial epicondyle as this is painful and is more likely to cause trophic skin changes.

The ulnar nerve lies just posterior to the medial epicondyle and is at risk from a misplaced injection.

 Lateral injection at the elbow

Indication

Tennis elbow (lateral epicondylitis).

Technique

Palpate the point of the lateral epicondyle and feel the fleshy substance of the extensor muscles anterior. The most tender area is often over the periosteum just anterior to the lateral epicondyle. However, the pathology is in the muscle and you should aim to inject into the flesh of the extensor muscle to a depth of 1 cm.

Use a combination of 2 ml of 1% lidocaine (lignocaine) mixed with **either**: 10–25 mg hydrocortisone acetate, **or** 5–10 mg triamcinolone, **or** 10–20 mg methyl-prednisolone.

Frequency

Every 4–6 weeks. If there is no benefit after two or three injections, then consider alternative treatment or referral.

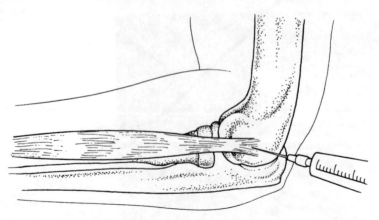

Figure 10.5   Lateral injection of the elbow

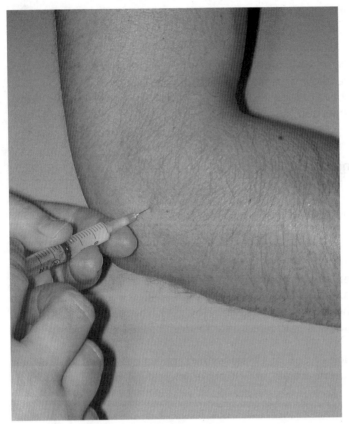

Figure 10.6   Injection for tennis elbow (lateral epicondylitis)

Structures at risk

Injection directly into bone or periosteum is exquisitely painful and should be avoided. Also injecting under pressure into the tendon has a theoretical risk of causing tendon damage.

Avoid injecting subcutaneously posterior to the lateral epicondyle as this may be painful and is more likely to cause trophic skin changes.

The radial nerve lies about 2 cm anterior and medial to the lateral epicondyle.

UPPER LIMB: HAND AND WRIST

 Injection of the base of the thumb

Indication

Arthritis of the carpometacarpal joint.

Technique

Palpate the extensor pollicis brevis and abductor pollicis longus tendons at the base of the thumb metacarpal. Next palpate the joint at the base of the metacarpal just anterior to these tendons. Insert a 21-gauge needle onto the metacarpal and 'walk' the needle into the joint. Insert to half a centimetre and inject gradually. Sometimes, gentle traction to the thumb is useful in gaining access to a very arthritic joint.

Use a combination of 2 ml of 1% lidocaine (lignocaine) mixed with **either:** 10–25 mg hydrocortisone acetate, **or** 5–10 mg triamcinolone, **or** 10–20 mg methyl-prednisolone.

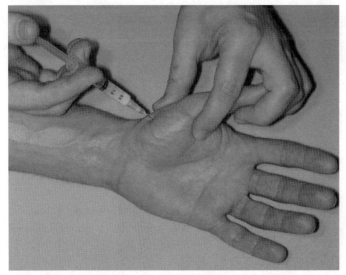

Figure 10.7   Injection of thumb carpometacarpal joint

Frequency

Every 4–6 weeks. If there is no benefit after two or three injections, then consider alternative treatment or referral.

Structures at risk

Injection directly into bone or periosteum is exquisitely painful and should be avoided.

Injection for De Quervain's tenosynovitis

Indication

Stenosing tenosynovitis of the abductor pollicis longus and extensor pollicis brevis tendons over the radial styloid.

Technique

Palpate the abductor pollicis longus and extensor pollicis brevis tendons over the dorsal aspect of the radial styloid. There is normally a thickened tendon sheath which is tender. As the thumb is moved, crepitus may be felt. Insert a 21-gauge needle in the line of the tendon into the tendon sheath to a depth of 3–5 mm and inject gradually.

   Use 1 ml of 10–25 mg hydrocortisone acetate.

Frequency

Every 4–6 weeks. If there is no benefit after two or three injections, then consider alternative treatment or referral.

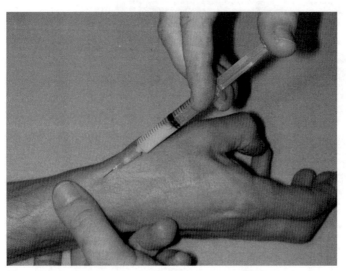

Figure 10.8   Injection for De Quervain's tenosynovitis

Structures at risk

Avoid injecting under pressure into the tendon as there is a theoretical risk of causing tendon damage. Subcutaneous injections may cause unsightly fat atrophy.

 ## Injection into the palm

Indication

Trigger finger or trigger thumb.

Technique

Palpate the nodule on the flexor tendon. This lies about 1 cm proximal to the level of the web space.

Insert a 21-gauge needle from proximal to distal just before the nodule. Passively flex and extend the finger a small amount to ensure the needle tip is in the tendon sheath not the tendon. If the needle moves, the tip is situated in the tendon and should be withdrawn a millimetre or two. This allows you to inject into the tendon sheath. Inject gradually and **do not** inject against resistance into the tendon.

Use a combination of 1 ml of 1% lidocaine (lignocaine) mixed with **either**: 10–25 mg hydrocortisone acetate, **or** 5–10 mg triamcinolone, **or** 10–20 mg methylprednisolone.

Frequency

Every 4–6 weeks. If there is no benefit after two injections then consider referral.

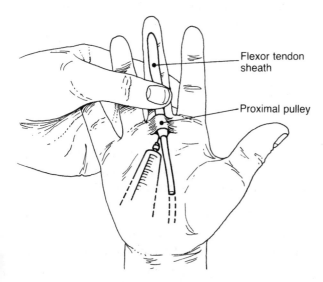

Flexor tendon sheath

Proximal pulley

Figure 10.9 Injection into the palm for trigger finger or thumb

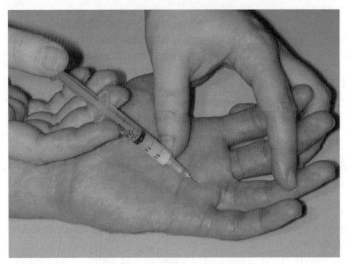

Figure 10.10 Injection into the palm for trigger finger

Structures at risk

Avoid injecting under pressure into tendon as there is a theoretical risk of causing tendon damage.

The digital nerves lie on either side of the tendon. Injection over the nodule and in line with the tendon is safe.

Injection of the carpal tunnel

This injection is not without serious risk and should only be carried out by a doctor experienced at performing it. Generally speaking it is less likely to be successful if the patient has had symptoms for more than 12 months.

Indication

Carpal tunnel syndrome.

Technique

Insert a 19-gauge needle just proximal to the distal wrist crease. This should be situated to the ulna side of the palmaris longus tendon and therefore not in the midline. Insert at an angle of 45 degrees until the needle is felt to pass through the flexor retinaculum. Then inject 1 ml of normal saline or local anaesthetic. If injection is resistance free and no pain or paraesthesia is experienced then inject 1 ml of 1% lidocaine (lignocaine) mixed with **either**: 10–25 mg hydrocortisone acetate, **or** 5–10 mg triamcinolone, **or** 10–20 mg methylprednisolone.

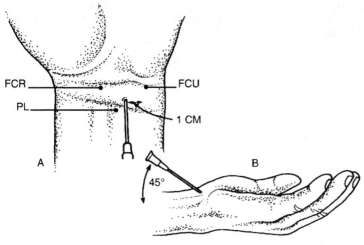

Figure 10.11   Injection of the carpal tunnel

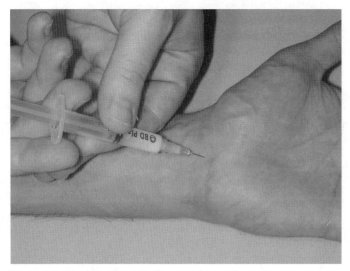

Figure 10.12   Injection into the carpal tunnel

Frequency

Once, then refer if no benefit.

Structures at risk

The median nerve is at risk. Stop injecting if any pain or paraesthesia radiates into the thumb or fingers. Steroid injection into the median nerve can cause permanent damage.

LOWER LIMB: HIP

Lateral injection to trochanteric bursa

Indication

Trochanteric bursitis.

Technique

With the patient lying on their side, palpate the greater trochanter. The point of maximum tenderness is usually just posterosuperior to the trochanter. Insert an 18-gauge needle and inject to a depth of 2–3 cm staying just lateral to the trochanter with the needle tip. Inject over a wide area.

Use a combination of 5 ml of 1% lidocaine (lignocaine) mixed with **either**: 10–25 mg hydrocortisone acetate, **or** 5–10 mg triamcinolone, **or** 10–20 mg methylprednisolone.

Frequency

Every 4–6 weeks. If there is no benefit after two injections then consider referral.

Structures at risk

Injection directly into bone or periosteum is exquisitely painful and should be avoided.

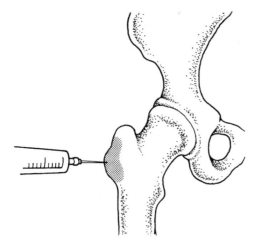

Figure 10.13 Injection of lateral aspect of hip

LOWER LIMB: KNEE

Lateral and medial injection of the knee

Indication

Arthritis and other intra-articular causes of pain.

Technique

This injection can be carried out from the lateral or the medial side but the lateral side is generally easier. With the patient supine and the leg relaxed palpate and move the patella from side to side. From the desired side insert an 18-gauge needle just posterior to the superior pole of the patella. Aim to pass the needle to almost its full depth between the patella and femur. This is made easier if an effusion is present. The effusion can also be aspirated confirming the intra-articular position of the needle before injecting. If there is no effusion, there should be no resistance to injection if the needle is correctly situated in the joint.

Use a combination of 5 ml of 1% lidocaine (lignocaine) mixed with **either**: 25–50 mg hydrocortisone acetate, **or** 20 mg triamcinolone, **or** 40 mg methylprednisolone.

Frequency

Every 4–6 weeks. If there is no benefit after two injections then consider referral.

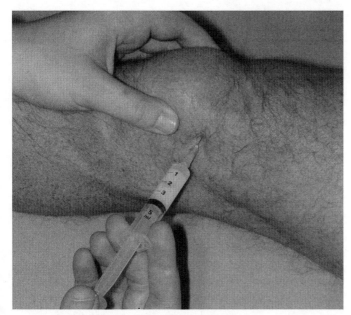

Figure 10.14   Lateral injection into knee joint

Structures at risk

Injection directly into bone or periosteum is exquisitely painful, so try and avoid it.

Lower limb: foot and ankle

The most common foot injection now undertaken in foot and ankle orthopaedic outpatients is an injection of a Morton's neuroma. This is usually carried out under ultrasound guidance and is therefore not discussed in this chapter.

Injection of the first metatarsophalangeal joint for hallux rigidus is no longer commonly performed. Treatment of this condition is with analgesia, orthotics or surgery.

Chapter **11**

Physiotherapy
Jane Moser

INTRODUCTION

Exercise in the treatment of musculoskeletal disorders is undervalued and underused. Patients are increasingly discontented with medication as a panacea and are seeking alternatives. Giving positive, specific advice and exercise has not only a physical effect but also a psychological one. Patients feel involved and can develop a sense of control and responsibility for their problem. What do you advise when you are confronted by a patient in a busy surgery? Do you feel that you have any positive advice for a patient with low back pain for example, or do you feel there is nothing you (or they) can do? Your attitude and behaviour (along with those of anyone the patient may come in contact with) will influence how a person will perceive and react to their musculoskeletal disorder. But you, as their doctor, definitely have an influence ('The doctor said …') which may be almost impossible to alter.

This chapter aims to give an overview of simple advice and exercises that can be shown to patients with orthopaedic problems. They are presented by regional areas of the body, as ordered in the earlier chapters (shoulder, elbow, wrist, cervical spine, lumbar spine, hip, knee, foot and ankle). Each area also has a section on general post-operative guidelines for common orthopaedic operations.

The exercises have been divided into programmes depending on the patient's predominant presentation. This approach is simplistic and limited to relatively straightforward orthopaedic problems. There is no one universal effective exercise for each area of the body. Exercises are selected as a result of assessment findings and the format used here attempts to guide you to appropriate exercises. Not all the exercises in a selected programme may be necessary and I envisage you will not have the time to show the patient more than two or three exercises. However, it is difficult to shorten the exercise programmes further without ignoring key movements or muscles that commonly need re-education in orthopaedics. Therefore, following your examination, choose the movement which appears the most functionally restrictive in terms of stiffness or weakness. Ideally only a few exercises (3–5 maximum) should be given and realistic goals set. This, combined with written information, will improve compliance. These programmes have been written for you, not for the patient. They can be viewed as a library and the information used to create patient information and exercise sheets if you wish.

These exercises can be regarded as 'first aid'. They have been selected because they:

- are relatively simple to teach and perform
- involve little or no equipment
- can be shown easily in a primary care setting.

Discrimination between sensations of unaccustomed exercise and the patient's presenting symptoms must be made. Sensations of stiffness, aching, stretching, tightness, tiredness can be regarded as normal, particularly if the patient has not done any recent activity or has had the problem a long time. However, as a general rule **pain should not progressively worsen** either during or after these exercises and this warning must be given. If pain/symptoms are worsening with the selected exercises:

- check that the exercise is being performed correctly
- reduce the number of repetitions and/or
- change the exercise (e.g. weight bearing to non-weight bearing)
- stop the exercises and reassess analgesia and management.

Although the exercises appear simple, sometimes patients need encouragement and help to do them and to do them correctly. Refer patients to a chartered physiotherapist if they:

- are not making progress with simple exercises
- require comprehensive rehabilitation
- have severe and/or complicated presentations.

Physiotherapy assessment involves a detailed analysis of the neuromuscular skeletal system and commonly lasts for 40 minutes. Attention will also be given to the patient's lifestyle, psychological status and motivation. Exercise is a core treatment modality but additional treatment techniques can also be given, such as:

- education and advice
- manual therapy (mobilizations, manipulation, soft tissue techniques)
- strapping and/or splintage
- electrotherapy.

Normally, 20–30 minute follow-up physiotherapy appointments will be given and will include feedback, reassessment and treatment. The simple exercises in this chapter are thus no substitute for assessment and treatment by a chartered physiotherapist where this is needed and patients who meet the above criteria above should be referred.

In this chapter, in addition to advice and exercises, each area of the body has a section on post-operative management following common orthopaedic surgery. Management will depend on:

- the type of surgical technique used
- the patient's general health and functional demands
- the surgeon's beliefs/attitude to rehabilitation
- the resources available.

Large differences in the post-operative management of patients may be found. These guidelines can only be general in nature and primarily represent local practice (Oxford), especially as there appears to be little literature concerning the effects of post-operative protocols. Specific queries regarding post-operative management of patients must be directed to the surgical unit.

Functional restrictions can be long term, despite intervention and patients may need help and require specific advice regarding adaptations. This can be obtained through occupational therapy departments (hospital or community) or through Disabled Living Centres (see Appendix 11.2).

SHOULDER

General advice for people with shoulder problems

If pain is experienced at night suggest:

- pillow/rolled towel under arm at night if lying on back, or
- pillows in front (like a bolster) if lying on pain-free side.

Shoulder exercises

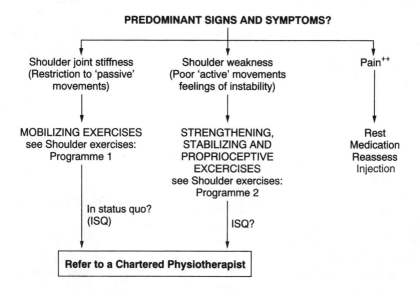

Shoulder mobilizing exercises

Shoulder programme 1

Signs and symptoms are predominantly joint stiffness.

Advice: It may be helpful to do these exercises after the application of local heat (e.g. warm bath, shower, hot water bottle – see Appendix 11.1).

Pendulum
Leaning forwards (with support if necessary)
Let arm hang down, relaxed
Swing arm
1. forward and back
2. side to side
3. round in circles (both ways)
Repeat 5–10 times each movement

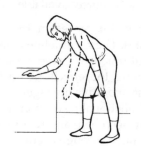

Scapula movements
Sitting, keep arms relaxed
Bring shoulders up and forwards
Then roll them 'down' and backwards
Repeat 5–10 times

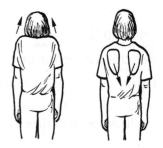

Assisted elevation in lying
Lying on back
Support arm with other hand at wrist
Lift arms overhead
Can start with elbows bent
Repeat 5–10 times

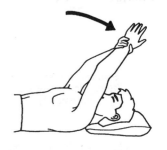

Lateral rotation
Sitting holding a stick (rolling pin, umbrella)
Keep affected side elbow into body throughout
Push with unaffected side, so hand of affected side is moving away from midline
Repeat 5–10 times
(Can be done lying down)

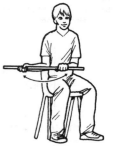

Hand behind back
Place hand behind body
Gently assist it with unaffected hand
Or use a towel/belt to pull it up back
Repeat 5–10 times

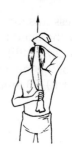

NB: This is often the last movement to return – do not force if painful (rather than stiff)

Shoulder strengthening and stabilizing exercises

Shoulder programme 2

Signs and symptoms are predominantly of weakness. Test and compare to the other side. What is weak?

Advice: Patients should not experience pain but they may feel muscle discomfort.

Lateral rotators: glenohumeral
Sit or stand
Elbow bent and close to body
Use other hand (or wall/doorway) to stop movement
Attempt to push affected wrist away from body
Keep elbow in
Do not let movement occur
Hold for 10 seconds
Repeat 10 times and build to 30
Progress this to using an elastic cord
Allow the hand to move outwards (keep elbow close still)
Control the movement out *and back in*
Repeat 10–30 times

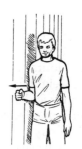

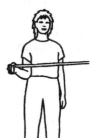

Medial rotators: glenohumeral
Sit or stand
Elbow bent and close to body
Use other hand (or wall/doorway) to stop movement
Attempt to pull wrist towards stomach
Do not let the movement occur
Hold for 10 seconds
Repeat 10 times and build to 30

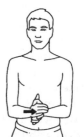

Progress this to using an elastic cord
Allow the hand to move inwards (keep
elbow close still)
Control the movement in *and back out*
Repeat 10–30 times

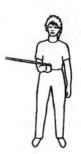

Scapula stabilization exercise
In sitting, standing, any position
Roll shoulder blade down and back gently
Do not arch the low back
Keep it there
Hold for 10 seconds
Repeat 10–30 times
Try and do this regularly through the day

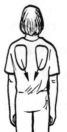

**Weight-bearing strengthening/
proprioception**
On all fours
Take weight forwards through arms
Then try and lift *unaffected* arm
Stretch unaffected arm in different
directions
Keep balance on affected arm,
with shoulder blade *flat* against
chest wall
Repeat 10 times

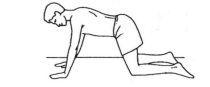

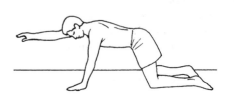

Post-operative management and advice

Shoulder replacement

These patients will be in hospital for approximately 5 days and will start
rehabilitation with the physiotherapist and occupational therapist. Outpatient physiotherapy is normally arranged for discharge and the patient will
have a home exercise programme.

Certain movements may be restricted for up to 3 months if soft tissue
reconstruction (e.g. rotator cuff repair or lengthening) has also been performed. The patient with a standard hemiarthroplasty or total shoulder
replacement can wean themselves out of the sling and attempt activities at
waist level as they feel able. Early movement should be encouraged. The
patient's ability to move the arm against gravity in the long term depends on

whether the rotator cuff is functional (it is often damaged and irreparable) and whether the joint movement previously was limited by soft tissue contracture. The main consistent post-operative outcome is pain relief.

Rough guidelines for return to functional activities are:

- Driving, sedentary or light work, swimming, gardening (light) – 6–8 weeks.
- Overhead activities/manual work – 3–6 months (perhaps never).

Most improvements are gained in the first 6 months, but improvements in strength and range of movement can continue for up to 18 months/2 years.

Manipulation under anaesthetic/arthroscopic release

These patients are normally day cases, but can stay overnight. Physiotherapy needs to be implemented immediately to retain movement gained at operation. Outpatient physiotherapy appointments must be arranged as priority.

Subacromial decompression

This operation is usually done by arthroscopy, as a day case. Although scars are small this operation can be painful in the first few days as a result of bony resection and ligament release. Heavy lifting is discouraged in the first week, but otherwise patients are encouraged to regain their shoulder movements as soon as possible. This is not normally a problem. They can return to normal activities as they feel able, where possible avoiding shoulder impingement positions (arm at shoulder height). Outpatient physiotherapy is often arranged.

Rotator cuff repair

Although patients may only be in hospital overnight following this procedure, this operation can have a considerable rehabilitation period. The extent and security of the reconstruction can vary enormously and has a direct bearing on the rehabilitation times and outcomes. Patients may be immobilized for up to 6 weeks in a sling (and in some units, a splint keeping the shoulder in abduction and external rotation). During this time the patients are normally given strict instructions on what to avoid and the joint may only be moved passively (no or minimal muscle contraction).

Once this initial period is over, the patient then embarks on a progressive exercise programme aimed at regaining muscle control and range of movement. Supervised rehabilitation is vital for these patients.

General guidelines for return to functional activities are:

- Driving – 5–9 weeks post-operatively.
- All lifting should be avoided for 3 months. Patients with overhead or manual work may be off for 6 months.

The greatest progress is seen in the first 6 months, but improvements, particularly in strength, can continue for 2 years.

ELBOW

General advice for elbow problems (particularly related to soft tissue/overuse, e.g. lateral and medial epicondylitis)

- *Encourage rest of the area*, therefore avoid repetitive wrist, forearm and gripping movements.
- For lateral epicondylitis, lifting must be done with *palm up* to reduce extensor activity.
- Local heat and/or cold may be helpful for pain relief (see Appendix 11.1 for details).
- *Temporary* use of splints for activity can be helpful. Counterforce (tennis elbow) braces are available from sports shops. 'Cock up' wrist splints can be helpful if the pain is severe (to enforce rest).
- If there are problems with sustained gripping activities; suggest change of grip size (e.g. enlarging diameter of pen size for writing) and also increase awareness to try and loosen grip to a minimum.

Elbow exercises

Many pains and discomforts around the elbow can be referred or influenced from the cervical spine. Worsening symptoms, particularly of paraesthesia, numbness or pain, should be viewed with caution and a reassessment of management made.

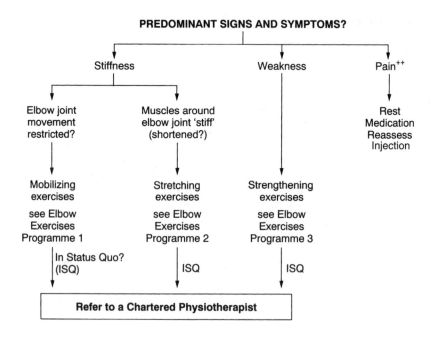

Elbow mobilizing exercises

Elbow programme 1

Predominant signs and symptoms are of elbow joint stiffness.

Flexion (with supination)

Lying on back, upper arm supported on
bed/floor
Bend hand towards shoulder, palm facing
Then straighten arm out
Repeat 5–10 times

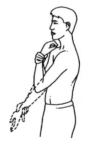

If weakness is not a problem this can be
done in standing or sitting
Can also add in forearm movements
Thumb towards shoulder (mid-range)
Back of hand towards shoulder (with
pronation)

Extension

In standing or lying
Keep elbow close to body
Straighten elbow as much as possible
(can have palm facing in front, behind or
into body)
Repeat 5–10 times

Supination

Standing or sitting
Elbow close to body and bent to 90 degrees
Turn forearm, so palm facing up to ceiling
Repeat 5–10 times
Can hold an end-weighted stick (e.g.
hammer) to add extra stretch

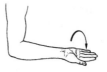

Pronation

As above but with palm facing down to floor
Can also add an end-weighted stick

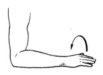

Elbow stretching exercises

Elbow programme 2

Predominant signs and symptoms are of elbow stiffness related to shortened
muscles.

Forearm extensors (tennis elbow)
Stand or sit
Straighten elbow (and keep it straight)
Curl fingers up into a fist
Then flex wrist
Hold for 20 seconds
Repeat 5 times

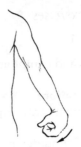

Forearm flexors (golfer's elbow)
Stand or sit
Link fingers together
Straighten elbow (and keep it straight)
Then extend wrist
Hold for 20 seconds
Repeat 5 times

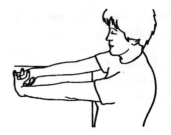

Elbow strengthening exercises

Elbow programme 3

Predominant signs and symptoms are weakness of the elbow.

Extension (A)
Lying on stomach
Upper arm resting on bed
Straighten arm out
Repeat 20–30 times
Progress by adding weight in hand

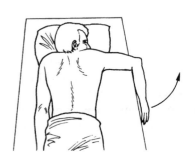

Extension (B)
Push-ups standing against wall
Progress to
1. push-ups from knees
2. push-ups from toes
Repeat 10–20 times

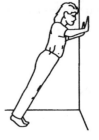

Flexion (and supination)
Stand or sit
Palm facing backwards
Bend elbow, palm towards shoulder
Repeat 20–30 times
Progress by adding a weight in hand

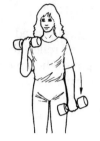

Pronation and supination (A)
Stand or sit
Elbow close to body and bent to 90-degree angle
Hold end-weighted stick (e.g. hammer)
Turn forearm so palm faces floor to ceiling
Keep control throughout the movement
Repeat 20–30 times

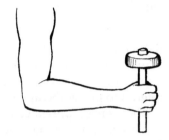

Pronation and supination (B)
Wringing action
Using a towel
Grip towel with hands
Twist arm in both directions
(palm up and palm down)

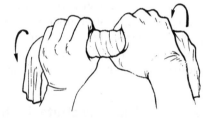

For forearm strengthening exercises, please see section on wrist strengthening exercises (Wrist programme 2).

Post-operative mangement and advice

Total elbow replacement

The rehabilitation starts as an inpatient, with input from both occupational therapists and physiotherapists. Assisted movements are commenced according to the surgeon's wishes (can start on day 1 or not until day 3). Early mobilization is encouraged but triceps repair needs protection for 6 weeks. Some centres use a removable posterior plaster of paris shell during this period, others discharge the patients after approximately 5 days with a sling and on-going exercise programme. Patients can gradually increase their functional activities as they are able. Most patients with this operation have rheumatoid arthritis, and the functional ability after this operation may be influenced by their other joint problems. Pain relief is the prime aim of replacement and there is often a residual flexion deformity that does not normally interfere with function. The prostheses are not designed for heavy or high levels of activity, and these are generally discouraged.

Tennis elbow release

The exact surgical procedure may vary for this operation and post-operative rehabilitation will reflect this. Some patients may attend as a day case and have no specific physiotherapy arranged (as in Oxford), while in other centres patients may have the elbow immobilized for 2 weeks and then follow a full rehabilitation programme over 8 weeks. Forearm support bands can continue to be used for working/leisure activities to reduce the possibility of recurrence.

WRIST AND HAND

Presentations of wrist and hand pain without injury or trauma can be an initial symptom, or part of 'non-specific' arm pain, often related to repetitive use at work or hobbies. This can lead to considerable disability with employment issues. Conservative care and positive strategies are indicated with early referral to physiotherapy if disability is high.

The exercises presented here are mainly for the wrist. The hand tends to exercise itself with everyday use. Following injury or trauma, especially involving damage to tendon or nerve, the hand requires specific rehabilitation under the supervision of the surgeon and therapy staff. Therefore hand exercises, other than general grip strengthening, have not been included. Giving advice on joint protection strategies, however, can be of considerable benefit to those with degenerative joint disease of the wrist and hand and some ideas are given. For more detailed advice and assessment refer to a hand or occupational therapist.

General advice and strategies for joint protection of the hand (e.g. for OA thumb carpometacarpal (CMC) and metacarpal phalangeal joints (MCP), OA or RA)

- Use tap turners (variety of models), electrical tin openers.
- When sustained gripping required, enlarge grip size to change the loading on the joints (e.g. on tools, pens, kitchen items).
- Local warmth may be helpful for pain relief. Warm water can be used. More heat can be given to the joint if rubber gloves protect the skin (see Appendix 11.1).
- If the hand feels weak, can advise patient to try exercising (general gripping action) against spongy material such as ready-made children's Playdough. (Or patients can make their own dough using 1 cup of water, 1 cup of flour, ½ cup of salt, 1 tablespoon of cooking oil, 1 teaspoon of cream of tartar, food colouring. Boil these together and keep in polythene bag. The putty can be used without taking it out of the bag.)

General advice for people with wrist problems

- Local heat and/or cold may be helpful for pain relief (see Appendix 11.1 for details).

- Wrist supports may be helpful (with the wrist held in some extension). Advise intermittent use at night (e.g. carpal tunnel) or during day (e.g. when involved in gripping or lifting activities). NB: Patients with De Quervain's tendonitis require thumb immobilization as well.

Wrist exercises

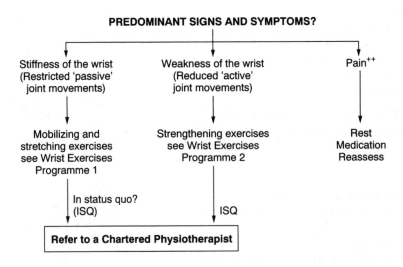

PREDOMINANT SIGNS AND SYMPTOMS?

Stiffness of the wrist (Restricted 'passive' joint movements)	Weakness of the wrist (Reduced 'active' joint movements)	Pain[++]
Mobilizing and stretching exercises see Wrist Exercises Programme 1	Strengthening exercises see Wrist Exercises Programme 2	Rest Medication Reassess

In status quo? (ISQ)   ISQ

Refer to a Chartered Physiotherapist

Mobilizing exercises for the wrist

Wrist programme 1

Predominant signs and symptoms are of stiffness in wrist.
    There is some overlap between the exercises for the elbow and wrist.

Advice: These exercises may be more comfortable after the application of local heat.

Extension (A)
Place hand and forearm flat on table/surface
Lift hand up in air
Keep forearm down
Repeat 5–10 times

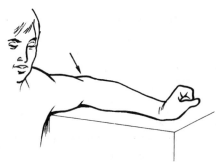

NB: If elbow extension is maintained throughout, the forearm flexors will be stretched

Extension (B)
Place elbows and palms of hands together
in front of body
Keep palms together
Take elbows apart
Repeat 5–10 times

Flexion
Place forearm on table, palm down
Place wrist crease on edge of table
Let hand drop over edge of table
Can add a stretch with other hand
Repeat 5–10 times

NB: If elbow extension is maintained
throughout, the forearm extensors will be
stretched

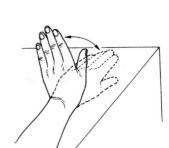

Radial and ulnar deviation
Place forearm and hand on table, palm
down
Keep forearm still
Slide hand from one side to other side
Repeat 5–10 times each side

Supination and pronation
Please see elbow exercises for description of exercises

Strengthening exercises for the wrist

Wrist programme 2

The predominant signs and symptoms are of weakness of the wrist.

Forearm extensors
Forearm resting on table, palm down
Wrist crease on edge of table, hand dropped
over edge of table
Lift hand up
Repeat 20–30 times

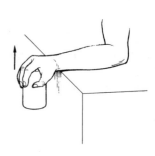

Progress by
1. adding ulnar and radial deviation
2. holding a weight
3. pulling against an elastic rope

Forearm flexors
Forearm resting on table, palm facing up
Wrist crease on edge of table, hand dropped
over edge
Lift hand up
Repeat 20–30 times
Progress by
1. adding ulnar and radial deviation
2. holding a weight
3. pulling against an elastic rope

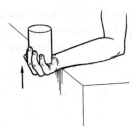

Post-operative management and advice

Carpal tunnel release

This procedure is done as a day case. Patients are discharged with a bulky bandage, maintained for 2 weeks. They are encouraged to resume daily activities as they are able and will not have outpatient physiotherapy arranged, unless they are experiencing problems in regaining function.
    Guidelines for return to activities are:

- Return to light work within 3–4 weeks.
- Return to heavy work 8–12 weeks.
- Grip strength and endurance may take 3–6 months or longer to achieve, and for some may remain incomplete.

Surgical release of Dupytren's contracture

This procedure is also done as a day case. Patients will be discharged with a bulky bandage +/− a plaster of paris backslab, which is maintained for 2–3 days (longer if a skin graft has been taken). If no skin graft is taken, patients are seen by a hand therapist around the third post-operative day to remove the bandage, commence mobilization and fit a splint. The splint is used to counteract the tendency for the surgical scar to contract during wound healing. Most patients wear the splint at night for 3 months (or longer) and some wear it during the day as well.
    Therapy aims to maintain the finger extension range gained from surgery and to restore pre-operative flexion. In a few cases, specific treatment modalities are required, e.g. ultrasound, serial splinting, silicone elastomer treatment.
    Guidelines for return to functional activities are:

- Return to desk job 2–6 weeks.
- Return to driving 2–4 weeks.
- Return to manual work 6–8 weeks.

CERVICAL SPINE

Neck pain and related symptoms into the arm, shoulder and head can be very frightening for patients and may lead to patterns of disability similar to those described in the Clinical Standards Advisory Group (1994) publication on back pain. Therefore reassurance combined with practical advice and early active treatment, particularly for patients who appear anxious or distressed, is advised.

For patients who have sustained a whiplash injury, there is a comprehensive patient education booklet based on research which deals with self-help and incorporates the psychosocial issues: *The Whiplash Book* (Stationery Office 2002, ISBN 011702029X; www.tso.co.uk/bookshop) is recommended and incorporates many of the advice strategies given below.

General advice for people with cervical spine problems

- Give these patients confidence and positive reassurance of their body's ability to recover. Be aware of language/labels (e.g. arthritis of the spine or whiplash) which might frighten patients and contribute to disability (e.g. 'The doctor says it is "wearing out" therefore I must use it less').

- Patients should be encouraged to remain physically active, with activities that they can manage. Advise them to increase activities progressively over a few days or weeks.

- Unloading the compression force through the spine can be helpful. Advise patients to use resting positions in lying, with the head supported with pillows so that it is comfortable. This can be no pillows for some people but those with nerve root symptoms often prefer two or more pillows.

- On the whole, collars are not recommended. Continuous and prolonged use of a collar should be discouraged and is associated with a poor prognosis following whiplash injuries. Collars can disturb balance for some patients and should not be worn when driving, as it may invalidate their car insurance policy. However, soft collars worn at night may be helpful.

- Changing positions regularly is recommended. Minimize sustained stooping postures. When sitting, it may be more comfortable to lean back and have head and neck supported. If sitting at a workstation or watching television, suggest the screen is straight ahead and at a comfortable height. Often the screen needs to be higher (e.g. on a box). The chair should have adequate *lumbar* spine support (can use rolled-up towel or cushion etc. – see lumbar spine advice).

- Attention to the pillow arrangement is indicated if pain is worse at night or on waking. It is often helpful if the depth of pillow is the distance from the shoulder to the side of the head. To support the neck, a rolled-up hand towel (or roll of foam) can be placed down the front of the pillowcase to give extra support (see Figure 11.8). This works best with a soft-top pillow.

- Avoiding sleeping on the stomach may also reduce symptoms.

- Heat pads or hot water bottles can be helpful on overactive muscles (often upper trapezius). 'Wheat bags' that can be heated in the microwave are

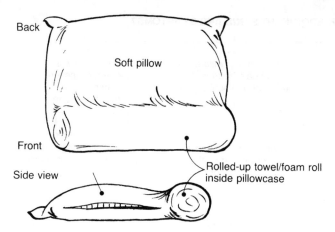

Figure 11.8 Support for cervical spine

Back

Soft pillow

Front

Side view

Rolled-up towel/foam roll inside pillowcase

useful as they are highly malleable. Cold (ice) packs can also be tried and local massage (see Appendix 11.1).

- Reduce stress levels as much as possible with the use of music, relaxation tapes, etc.

Cervical spine exercises

In clinical practice, exercises that increase symptoms (pain or paresthesiae) *away* from the cervical area often appear to be unhelpful. As a guide, with exercise, pain/paraesthesiae **should not peripheralize** – i.e. pain becomes more prominent away from the cervical area (into head, scapula, shoulders, arm and/or hands) – even if the cervical pain is resolving. If the patient has arm pain, check for and monitor any neurological signs.

Cervical spine presentations have been divided roughly into two categories. Firstly those with localized neck pain, secondly those with referred pain into the head, scapula, shoulder or arm. The presentations can be extremely varied in terms of severity and irritability (e.g. how easy it is to exacerbate symptoms and how long they take to settle) and to reflect this they have been further divided.

Moderate or severe nerve root pain requires individual assessment and treatment with close monitoring of neurological signs and symptoms. For those with mild symptoms, advise exercises, but with instructions to seek help if symptoms deteriorate. Be cautious of patients who present with minimal or moderate symptoms but whose head and shoulders are in abnormal postures (e.g. head sideflexed and/or rotated). The postures are commonly antalgic and movements reversing them can significantly worsen symptoms. Refer these cases to a chartered physiotherapist for individual assessment.

If specific exercises are not helpful, continue to encourage general movement and gentle activity such as walking, movement in a pool, trunk rotations and arm movements. This helps reduce fear and disability.

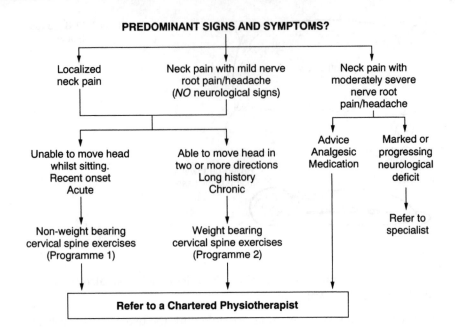

PREDOMINANT SIGNS AND SYMPTOMS?

Localized neck pain

Neck pain with mild nerve root pain/headache (*NO* neurological signs)

Neck pain with moderately severe nerve root pain/headache

Unable to move head whilst sitting. Recent onset Acute

Able to move head in two or more directions Long history Chronic

Advice Analgesic Medication

Marked or progressing neurological deficit

Non-weight bearing cervical spine exercises (Programme 1)

Weight bearing cervical spine exercises (Programme 2)

Refer to specialist

Refer to a Chartered Physiotherapist

Cervical spine exercises

Cervical spine programme 1

The predominant symptoms are local cervical spine pain and/or mild arm symptoms without neurological changes with **recent onset symptoms (i.e.'acute')**. They may have severe limitation of movement (only move in one or two directions) in sitting or standing (antigravity postures).

NB: All these exercises are designed to improve movement and ease pain. As a guide, pain and/or paraesthesiae should not move away from the neck (see above). If an exercise aggravates pain, advise patients to reduce repetitions and/or range before discontinuing that particular exercise. They should continue with other exercises and general advice strategies.

Non-weight-bearing exercises
- These exercises should be done in a comfortable starting position if possible.
- This may require one or more pillows which can be gradually reduced until head is resting on floor/bed.
- A heat pad can also be used at the same time.
- The exercises can be done 20–30 minutes after appropriate medication.

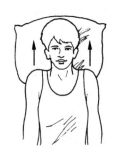

Shoulder shrug in lying
Gently raise shoulders up towards ears
Try and get both sides to move smoothly

Then let them relax
Repeat 5–10 times

Upper cervical flexion, lower cervical extension in lying 'chin tucks'

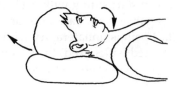

Keep head *supported* on pillow/floor *throughout* the movement
Tuck chin in
Pressing back of neck towards pillow/floor
It is like a small nodding movement
A stretch is normally felt at the back of the neck
(do not clench teeth during this)
Repeat 5–10 times

Cervical rotations in lying

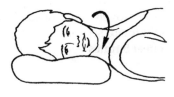

Keep head *supported* on pillow/floor *throughout* the movement
Try and keep chin tucked in as in exercise above
Turn head, so looking to side
Return to midline
Repeat 5 times to one side, then repeat to other side

(Can progress onto cervical spine exercise programme 2 when confident to do so)

Cervical spine exercises

Cervical spine programme 2

Exercises for patients with local cervical spine pain and/or mild arm symptoms without neurological changes with **insidious onset and long-term symptoms (i.e.'chronic')**

NB: All these exercises are designed to improve movement and ease pain. As a guide, pain and/or paraesthesiae should not move away from the neck (see above). If an exercise aggravates pain, advise patients to reduce repetitions and/or range before discontinuing that particular exercise. They should continue with other exercises and general advice strategies.

Weight-bearing exercises
If they are unable to do these, go to cervical spine exercises in programme 1.

Upper cervical flexion, lower cervical extension in sitting 'chin tucks'

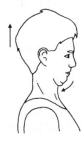

Sitting in a firm (and high) backed chair
Look straight ahead
Pull chin in
Lift crown of head up
Feel stretch at back of neck
Do not let chin drop down (so head is forward)

Repeat 5–10 times
Modifications:
1. can start sitting with back and head resting against wall/back of door
2. if pain is unilateral try with head slightly tilted (sideflexed) to one side
3. progress exercise by adding manual pressure on the chin

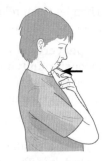

For strength:
Maintain chin tuck position
Place hand on forehead
Resist movement of head forwards
Hold for 10 seconds
Repeat 5 times

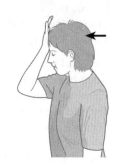

Cervical rotation (discontinue if dizzy or light-headed)
Sitting upright
Try and keep chin gently pulled in (as above)
Turn head to one side
Aim to get chin over shoulder
Repeat 5 times to one side, then repeat to other side

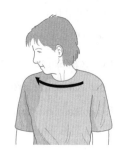

For strength:
Resist movement with hand
Hold for 10 seconds
Repeat 5 times
Repeat to the other side

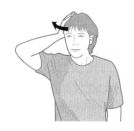

Cervical side flexion (discontinue if dizzy or light-headed)
Sitting upright
Try and keep chin gently pulled in (as above)
Look straight ahead
Tilt ear towards shoulder

(often will feel stretch on opposite side)
Repeat 5 times to one side, then repeat to other side

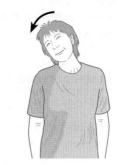

For strength:
Resist movement with hand
Hold for 10 seconds
Repeat 5 times
Repeat to the other side

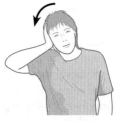

Cervical extension (discontinue if dizzy or
    light-headed)
Sitting upright
Do first exercise in this programme
Then, at finishing point, look up at ceiling
Start by giving support at back of head with fingers
Try and keep chin tucked in on return to
starting position
Repeat 5–10 times

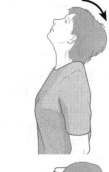

For strength:
Resist movement with hand
Hold for 10 seconds
Repeat 5 times

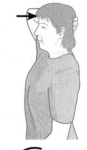

Cervical spine 'stretch'
Sitting upright
Place clenched fist between chin and chest
Put other hand behind head
Gently pull head forward and down
Feel stretch at back of neck
Repeat 5–10 times

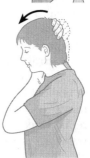

(may need to put a book or folded towel under 'clenched' hand to affect the upper cervical spine)

Post-operative management and advice

Anterior cervical decompression and fusion

This operation may be performed by either an orthopaedic surgeon or a neuro-surgeon. The use of collars routinely in post-operative care has not been established. They may not be given at all or given for comfort, intermittent use or for more consistent use. Therefore check local protocols. Firm or soft collars can be used during the day (e.g. travelling), with a soft collar used at night. Outpatient physiotherapy may not be instigated, with patients given encouragement by the surgeons and staff to regain neck movements and general activities gradually. Neck movements should be re-established within 3 months, with minimal restriction for those who have had a single level fusion. Often, however, it is arm pain, sensory changes and motor weakness in arms and/or legs that are of prime concern in terms of outcome. However, if a patient appears to be very frightened regarding neck movements and does not appear to be progressing with self-directed rehabilitation, consider referral to physiotherapy.

Guidelines for return to functional activities are:

- Return to light work – 4–6 weeks.
- Return to driving – 4–6 weeks unless hard collar is worn (see previous advice on collar and driving).
- Avoid lifting completely for 6 weeks and then start with light items.
- Return to heavy work – 6–12 weeks.

LUMBAR SPINE

Diagnostic triage of patients with LBP should aim to identify possible serious spinal pathology (see lumbar spine chapter), which is excluded from the algorithm below. Criteria for triage and evidence-based management options of back pain are published as Clinical Guidelines, by the Royal College of General Practitioners (www.rcgp.org.uk).

The emphasis is on managing LBP, to reduce disability. Encouragement of normal activities, including an early return to work, even though patients may not be pain-free, is paramount. The presence of certain psychosocial factors, 'yellow-flags' (e.g. distress, 'fear avoidance' behaviours, etc.) may expedite referral to rehabilitation.

Simple advice aiming to reduce disability and promote self-help, given in booklet form, has been shown to have a positive effect on patients presenting with LBP in primary care. The *Back Book* has been updated and republished in 2002 (*The Back Book*, Stationery Office, London, ISBN 0117029505. www.tso.co.uk/bookshop). It is recommended.

General advice for people with lumbar spine problems

- Give them confidence and positive reassurance of natural history and that the back has a good ability to recover.
- Beware of using frightening language/labels such as 'arthritis of the spine'.
- Patients should be encouraged to remain physically active with activities that they can manage. Advise them to increase activities progressively over a few days or weeks. Promotion of improving general fitness is very useful. Patients often respond positively to this approach as they commonly feel they were unfit prior to their back pain episode.
- *Prolonged bed rest* (over 3 days) is *not* advised. It should not be viewed as a 'treatment'.
- Sitting is often problematic except for patients with spinal stenosis. Encourage a variety of postures to explore what is comfortable. Sitting postures can be altered by perching on the edge of seats/chairs, placing a rolled-up towel or cushion in the small of the back or using a wedge (see Figure 11.11).
- Changing positions regularly is recommended. Discourage long periods of inactivity and minimize sustained stooping postures and lifting.
- If having problems with sleep, it may help to try and firm-up soft mattresses/beds. In addition, when in side lying a rolled-up towel in the waist or pillow between legs can help.
- Heat pads or hot water bottles can be helpful. 'Wheat bags' that can be heated in the microwave are useful. Cold (ice) packs can also be tried and local massage. (See Appendix 11.1).
- Reduce stress levels as much as possible with use of music, relaxation tapes, etc.
- Fowler's rest position (Figure 11.12) is often helpful. It places the spine in a neutral, unloaded position.
- Encourage early return to work, even though they may not be pain-free. Can you liaise with employers in a positive way (graduated return or lighter duties)?

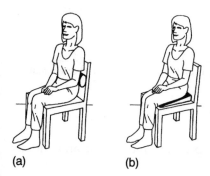

(a)   (b)

Figure 11.11 Sitting postures (a) using a lumbar roll; (b) using a wedge

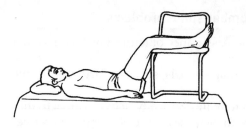

Figure 11.12   Fowler's resting position

Lumbar spine exercises

- As recommended by the Clinical Standards Advisory Group, the category of *mechanical* low back pain can be divided into simple backache and nerve root pain (see lumbar spine chapter for clinical criteria).These exercises can be applied to patients with simple backache and those with mild nerve root pain. If they have leg pain, check and monitor neurological signs.
- As a basic rule, **pain should not progressively worsen, either during or after these exercises**. In particular pain and/or paraesthesiae should not develop or worsen in the leg.
- If specific exercises are not helpful, continue to encourage improvement in their general fitness, e.g. walking, step-ups, gentle swimming and movements in a pool. This helps reduce fear and disability.
- People with nerve root signs, in 'distress', with a high level of disability or a number of yellow flags, may require early referral to a chartered physiotherapist for an individual assessment.

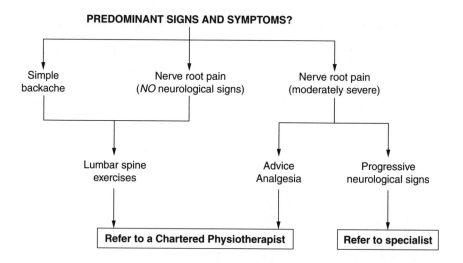

Lumbar spine programme

The exercises presented are general and promote movement and muscle activity around the trunk.

Movements in prone kneeling

On all fours
Tighten stomach muscles to flex or round back
Keep elbows straight and arms still
Then
1. let back extend or 'hollow'
2. move hips from side to side, 'wagging tail'
Repeat 10 times each

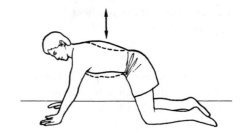

Pelvic tilting (in crook lying)

Lie with knees bent, feet flat on floor/bed
Tighten low stomach muscles (flatten them)
Try and press back towards floor/bed
Rocking pelvis backwards
Do not use feet to push!
Hold for 20 seconds, breathe easily
Repeat 10–15 times

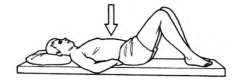

Bridging (in crook lying)

Lie with knees bent, feet flat on floor/bed
Tighten low stomach muscles (flatten them)
Try and press back into floor/bed
Then lift bottom up in air
Hold for 20 seconds, breathe easily
Repeat 10–15 times

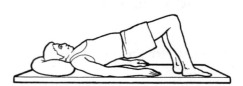

Flexion in lying

Lying on back
Take one knee up onto chest
Hug it with arms, pulling knee up towards nose
Repeat with other knee

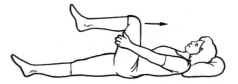

Try with both knees to chest
Repeat 10 times

'Passive' extension (in prone lying)

If the patient is unable to tolerate this,
can start with simply lying with
pillows under hips/lower abdomen
Lying on stomach
Hands under shoulder as if doing a
press-up
Keep back muscles relaxed
Push through arms, straightening elbows
Keep the hips and pelvis down
Feel back arching
Breathe out to get extra stretch
Repeat 10 times regularly if helpful

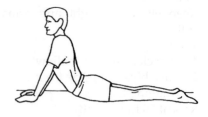

Extension (in standing)

Standing with hands on hips
Keep knees straight
Lean back
Do not let hips move forwards
Repeat 10 times regularly
(although easier to do in standing,
many prefer lying option)

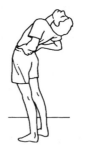

Flexion stretch (in prone kneeling)

On all fours
Keep hands stretched out in front
Sit back on heels
Let shoulders lower towards floor/bed
Hold for 5 seconds
Repeat 5 times

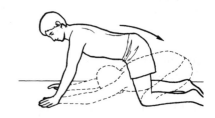

Pelvic tilting (in standing)

Stand with back against wall
Heels 10 cm away
Feet shoulder width apart
Tighten low stomach muscles
Try and move low back so it is touching
the wall
Repeat 10 times

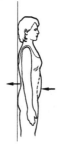

Post-operative management and advice

Lumbar surgery may be undertaken by either a neurosurgeon or an orthopaedic surgeon. This may also introduce a further variable in the post-operative management.

Lumbar discectomy

As with many orthopaedic procedures, there are now shorter inpatient stays (2–4 days) and quicker rehabilitation following surgery. Patients may be seen by a physiotherapist (and possibly an occupational therapist) while in hospital and given advice, education and a simple home exercise programme. Generally activity is encouraged, for example walking as much as possible, increasing the distance covered. Swimming may be started once the wound is healed.

Sitting is often uncomfortable and may be restricted initially. Patients can be advised to perch, sit in higher chairs and use a cushion, towel or roll of foam in the low back. Sitting times can be gradually increased. Driving may not be possible for 6 weeks and is dependent on sitting tolerance, pain response and flexibility of knee extension in sitting. Lifting is restricted commonly for several weeks (e.g. 8–12 weeks). For those unable to avoid it altogether (i.e. those with small children) guidelines should have been given regarding lifting techniques (the most important being to keep objects close).

Outpatient physiotherapy appointments may be made by the hospital staff on discharge or this may be initiated by the doctors when the patient is reviewed in an outpatient clinic. Routine outpatient physiotherapy may not be given. If a patient appears to be distressed or not gradually regaining activity, seek advice from the hospital (surgeon or physiotherapist) who may suggest that referral to a physiotherapist is indicated to supervise rehabilitation.

Lumbar decompression

The surgery involved in this procedure can vary considerably in its extent of bony resection. Rehabilitation may reflect this. Generally the principles of early mobilization and improving general fitness will be followed as with the discectomies. Greater emphasis may be placed on abdominal control and lumbar flexion range. Milestones of return to functional activities are as for patients following discectomy.

Spinal fusion

The post-operative care of these patients is similar to other spinal surgery, as above, but spinal movements are not encouraged excessively during the first 3 months of rehabilitation while the bone grafts are healing and the fusion is not biologically sound. The home exercise programme will emphasize muscle stabilizing work (abdominals, deep back extensors and gluteals).

Lifting should be avoided for the first 3 months and restriction on sitting (see above in section on lumbar discectomy) is also advised. However, walking and swimming can be encouraged as above.

Outpatient physiotherapy to progress the exercise programme may be organized for 6 weeks or thereafter by hospital staff or doctors in outpatient clinics.

Chemonucleolysis

This operation involves an injection of an enzyme (chymopapain) into the nucleus of the disc in the treatment of a disc prolapse (if the disc is not sequestrated). It is normally done as day surgery. Again prolonged sitting and lifting are not encouraged, particularly in the first 6 weeks.

HIP

General advice for people with hip problems

- Keep the joint moving but without stressing it, e.g. avoid unnecessary lifting, stairs, squatting, twisting and turning activities.
- Try swimming or movements in water.
- Try static cycling (seat may need to be raised).
- Raise seat heights and when getting out of chairs, use hands to push up with.
- Use a walking aid (stick or crutches) if unable to put all the weight through leg. Use a stick in the *opposite* hand. Try and walk as normally as possible with the walking aid.

Hip exercises

Be aware that buttock pain can be referred from the lumbar spine.

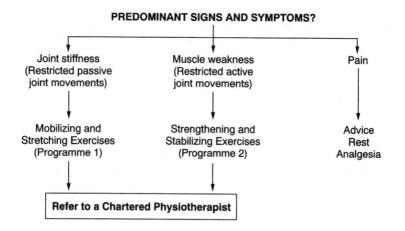

Mobilizing exercises for the hip

Hip programme 1

For predominant signs and symptoms of stiffness of the hip joint.

   Advice: It may be useful to do these after application of local heat (e.g. warm bath/shower, see Appendix 11.1).

Hip flexion in lying
Lying on back, legs out straight
Bend knee up towards chest
Return to start position
Repeat 5–10 times

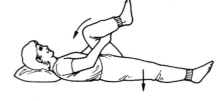

Hip flexion in standing
Stand facing a step (book or telephone directory if step is too high)
Place foot up onto step
Keep trunk still
Return to starting position
Gradually place foot on higher surface (use a stool/chair)
Repeat 5–10 times

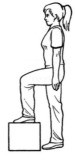

Hip extension in lying
Bend both knees up towards chest
Hug *unaffected* knee with hands (keep the pressure on)
Straighten out affected leg
May feel stretch in front of hip
This can be done on edge of table/bed to get more stretch
Repeat 5 times

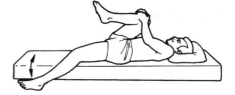

Hip extension in prone lying
Lie on stomach
Try and get front of hips in contact with bed/floor
(may need to start with small pillow or towel)
Tighten buttock muscles
Hold for 10 seconds

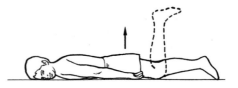

Repeat 10 times
1. Try and rest in this position
   for 15–20 minutes
2. Try and bend knee, keeping hips
   down into bed/floor
3. Can then add knee lift (see hip
   strengthening programme 2)

Medial rotation in prone lying
Lie on stomach
Bend knee to 90-degree angle
Keep knee still but let foot fall out to
side (away from other leg)
Repeat 5–10 times

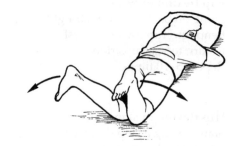

Abduction and external rotation
Lie on back, knees bent up, feet
on bed/floor
Let knees separate, keeping feet
together
Do not let back arch
Repeat 5–10 times

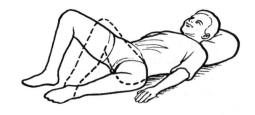

Strengthening exercises for the hip

Hip programme 2

For predominant signs and symptoms of weakness and instability around the
hip joint.

   Advice: Where possible use the weight-bearing exercises as they are more
functionally relevant and easier to practise.

Non-weight-bearing exercises
Bridging
Lie on back, knees bent up, feet on
bed/floor
Flatten back towards bed/floor
Lift buttocks off the bed/floor
Repeat 20–30 times

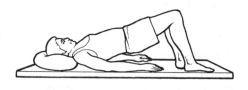

Progress to
1. lifting *unaffected* other foot off bed/floor
2. pushing up through affected leg alone

Extension in prone lying

Lying on stomach, knee bent to
90-degree angle
Lift knee 1 cm off bed / floor
Do not let back overarch
Repeat 20–30 times

NB: If unable to do this, start
with knee straight

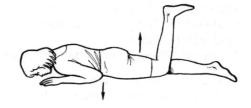

Weight-bearing exercises
Sit to standing

Sit on high surface (stool or
arm of sofa or armchair)
Keep affected leg back, other
leg slightly forward
Cross arms and try and
stand up
Then sit down slowly
Repeat 20–30 times
Progress by lowering the
height of the seat to a
normal chair
Further progress by lifting
unaffected leg off ground

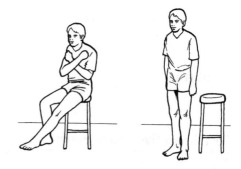

Step-ups

Step up onto a step using
your affected leg
Start with a small step (e.g.
telephone directory)
Gradually increase depth
of step
Repeat (aim for) 20–30 times

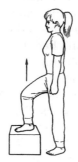

Dynamic alignment work in standing

This aims to retrain muscle control
and balance. It may also stretch
the calf.
Stand with feet hip width apart
Keep body upright
Bend knees fairly slowly, making sure
knees are moving over 2nd toe

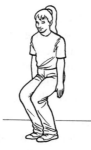

Keep heels on the ground
Start with small dips and increase
gradually (without pain)
Repeat 10–15 times, once a day minimum

Progress further by
1. doing on one leg, maintaining balance
2. stepping down off a small step
   (heel will come off ground for this)
3. increasing the depth of the step

Balance
Practise standing on one leg

Progress by
1. closing eyes
2. onto tiptoe

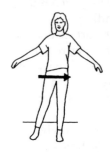

Post-operative management and advice

Total hip replacement

These patients are commonly in hospital for 5–7 days. This length of stay may reduce further with early supported discharge, where rehabilitation is given in the community. Most hip replacements are cemented and patients can weight bear as tolerated and leave hospital when at a safe functional level with a good gait pattern using crutches or two sticks. Patients are assessed by the occupational therapy team and given seat raises, helping hands (to avoid bending to floor level) and bath boards as necessary. They are not normally given outpatient physiotherapy appointments, but encouraged to increase their activity levels as able.

Precautions need to be taken for the first 3 months. Patients should avoid hip flexion (over 90-degree angle), particularly combined with adduction (e.g. sitting crossed legged, bending forward and lying on their non-operated side with the top leg unsupported). Patients are advised to sleep on their backs with a pillow between their legs for 6 weeks, after which time they can lie as they find comfortable.

Other than these restrictions, patients are encouraged to gradually increase their activity, especially walking. If the patient continues to have a poor gait pattern, referral to physiotherapy may be indicated. Poor gait is often due to disuse atrophy of the gluteal muscles and may require strengthening work (see strengthening hip exercises programme 2).

Guidelines for return to other functional activities are:

- Driving after 6–8 weeks.
- Return to desk job after 6–10 weeks.

- Return to manual work – 6 months, possibly never.
- Swimming can be started as soon as the wound is healed but breast stroke should be avoided for the first 6 weeks.
- Cycling can commence once sufficient range of motion is available, but the seat may need to be raised so that the hip is not flexing over 90 degrees.
- Gardening may not be possible for 3–4 months.
- Patients with uncemented hip replacements may have restricted weight bearing for 6–12 weeks but otherwise follow a similar (but slower) post-operative regime as described above.

KNEE

General advice for people with knee problems

- Avoid activities which increase swelling and/or pain (swelling will result in reflex inhibition of quadriceps, irrespective of the presence of pain).
- Keep the joint moving but without stressing it, e.g. avoid unnecessary lifting, stairs, squatting, kneeling, uneven ground, twisting and turning activities.
- Try static cycling (put the seat up high if movement is limited).
- Try swimming (freestyle legs may be more comfortable than breast stroke legs if there is lateral instability).
- Local heat and/or cold may be helpful (see Appendix 11.1 for details).
- Raise seat heights and use hands to push up with when getting out of chairs.
- Use a walking aid (stick or crutches) if unable to put all the weight through leg. Use a stick in the *opposite* hand. Try and walk as normally as possible with the walking aid.

Knee exercises

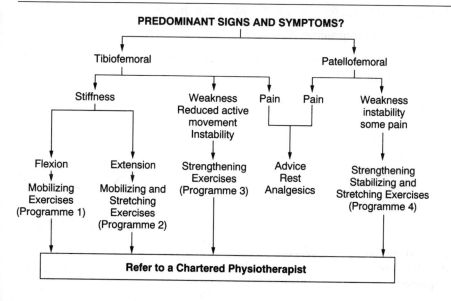

Mobilizing exercises for the knee (tibiofemoral joint)

Knee exercises programme 1

For patients with predominant signs and symptoms of *stiffness* of the tibiofemoral joint into *flexion*.

Knee flexion in sitting
Sit on a chair/table so can
get foot underneath
Bend knee, taking foot under
chair as far as possible
Straighten knee out
Start with a small range of
movement and gradually increase
Repeat 5–10 times

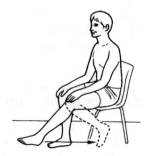

Knee flexion in prone lying
Lying on stomach, legs together
Bend knee as far as possible
Do not let hips rise
May feel stretch in front of thigh
or hip
Can give overpressure using the
other leg or use a towel around ankle
Repeat 5–10 times

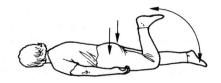

Mobilizing exercises for the knee (tibiofemoral joint)

Knee exercises programme 2

For patients with predominant signs and symptoms of *stiffness* of the tibiofemoral joint into *extension*.

Knee extension in sitting
Sit on a chair/table
Lean back, recline
Straighten knee out as far as possible
Start with a small range of movement
and gradually increase
Repeat 5–10 times

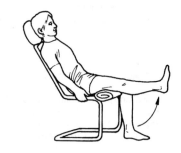

Knee extension in sitting/lying
Sit reclined back or lie on back with leg
supported

Place small towel under heel
Let gravity stretch joint into
extension
Can add hand pressure to give
extra stretch
Try and rest in this position for
several minutes
Increase to 10–15 minutes

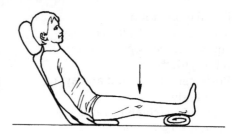

Strengthening exercises for the knee (tibiofemoral joint)

Knee exercises programme 3

For patients with predominant signs and symptoms of *weakness and instability*.
   NB: Straight leg raising is not helpful; it mainly exercises the hip flexors.
   The programme is divided into weight-bearing and non-weight-bearing
exercises. Weight bearing exercises should be used as long as there is no
increase in pain or swelling as they are more functionally relevant and easy to
practise in everyday life.

Non-weight-bearing exercises
Static quadriceps
If unable to do this try inner
range exercises
Half lying (e.g. propped up on
elbows)
Pull foot up
Push knee down into bed/floor
Try and raise heel (but keep knee
down)
Hold for 5 seconds and relax
Repeat (aim for) 20–30 times

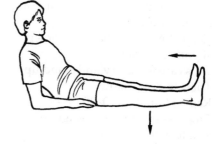

Inner range quadriceps
Half lying (propped up)
Rolled up towel under knee
Pull toes up towards you
Straighten leg
Keep knee down on towel
Hold for 5 seconds
Repeat (aim for) 20–30 times

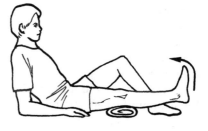

Static quadriceps/gluteals/adductors
Sitting with folded pillow or football
between knees

Feet flat on ground
Knees bent *less than* 90 degrees
Squeeze knees together (into
pillow/football)
Push feet into ground and away
from body
Feel and see thigh muscles tighten
Hold for 5 seconds
Repeat 20–30 times

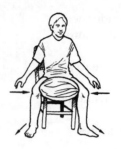

Progress by adding
1. buttock squeeze
2. lifting opposite buttock off chair

Weight-bearing exercises
These *must be pain-free* and not result in increased swelling.

Sit to standing

Sit on a high surface (stool or arm
of sofa or armchair)
Keep affected leg back, other leg
slightly forward
Cross arms and try and stand up
Then sit down slowly
Repeat (aim for) 20–30 times
Progress by lowering height of
seat to a normal chair
Further progress by lifting
unaffected leg off ground

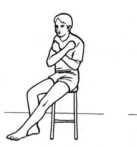
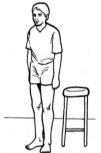

Step ups

Step up onto a step using your
affected leg
Start with a small step (e.g.
telephone directory)
Gradually increase depth of step
Repeat (aim for) 20–30 times

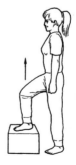

Dynamic alignment work in standing

This aims to retrain muscle control and
balance. It may also stretch the calf.
Stand with feet hip-width apart

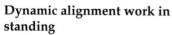

Keep body upright
Bend knees fairly slowly, making
sure knees are moving over 2nd
toe. When looking down inside
knees, should see big toes
Keep heels on the ground
Start with small dips and increase
gradually (without pain)
Repeat 10–15 times, once a day minimum

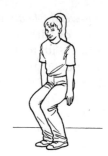

Progress further by
1. doing on one leg, maintaining balance
2. stepping down off a small step
   (heel will come off ground for this)
3. increasing the depth of the step

Hamstring strength and proprioception
Standing, hold on for support
Bend knee, lifting heel towards buttocks
Move it over a small distance, up and down
Then stop it suddenly
Repeat in different amounts of knee bend
Progress by adding weight at ankle
Repeat (aim for) 3–10 sets of 10
repetitions or until fatigued

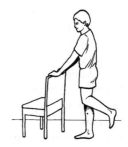

Balance
Practise standing on one leg
Progress onto tiptoe
Repeat with
1. eyes closeds
2. on tiptoes

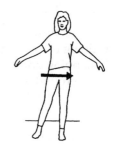

Exercises for patellofemoral symptoms

Knee exercises programme 4

Advice: Avoid squatting down and sustained weight-bearing activities on a
bent knee.
  Give stretches if muscles shortened on symptomatic side, otherwise start
on dynamic alignment exercise and sitting against the wall.
  NB: These exercises should be *pain-free*, but may feel tight, stretched, tired
or wobbly.

Non-weight-bearing exercise
Static quadriceps/gluteals/adductors
Sitting with folded pillow or football between knees
Feet flat on ground
Knees bent *less than* 90 degrees
Squeeze knees together (into pillow/football)
Push feet into ground and away from body
Feel and see thigh muscles tighten
Hold for 5 seconds
Repeat 20–30 times

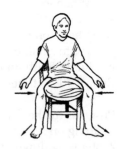

Progress by adding
1. buttock squeeze
2. lifting opposite buttock off chair

Weight-bearing exercises
Dynamic alignment work in standing
This aims to retrain muscle control and
balance. It may also stretch the calf.
Stand with feet hip-width apart
Keep body upright
Bend knees fairly slowly, making sure knees
are moving over 2nd toe. When looking
down inside knees, should see
big toes
Keep heels on the ground
Start with small dips and increase
gradually (without pain)
Repeat 10–15 times, once a day minimum

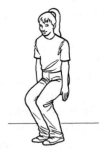

Progress further by
1. doing on one leg, maintaining balance
2. stepping down off a small step (heel will come
   off ground for this)
3. increasing the depth of the step

Sit against wall
Stand with back and heels against wall
Take three heel-to-toe steps forward,
keeping back against wall (this is important)
Slide back down wall, so sitting with
knees at approximately 60 degrees off full
extension
Hold for 10 seconds
Repeat 10–20 times
Then try and maintain position for 3 minutes

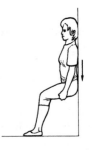

Hamstring stretches
NB: If symptoms of pain or
paraesthesiae occur into calf/foot,
discontinue and reassess.
Lying on back
Link arms around back of thigh
Straighten knee
Feel pull in back of thigh, buttock
or knee
Hold for 20 seconds
Repeat 5 times

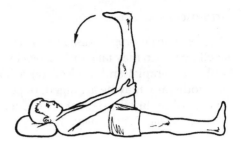

Calf stretch (gastrocnemius)
Stand with affected leg back in a
walking position
Lean forwards (can use chair/wall
for support)
Keep the back leg straight, heel
on ground
Feel the stretch in calf
Hold 20 seconds
Repeat 5 times

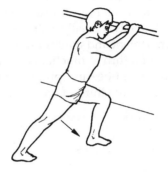

Post-operative management and advice

Total knee replacement (TKR)

Patients are advised to avoid contact or repetitive jarring sports. However, apart from this, there are no specific contraindications in terms of what patients can or cannot do following this operation, including kneeling.

As with the hip replacements there are initiatives to shorten inpatient stays with supported discharge care given in the community. At present routine discharge occurs after 5 days, once they have adequate knee flexion and are functionally safe and able. The patient will have a home exercise programme to continue with and outpatient physiotherapy is organized if deemed necessary. Patients appear to have to work harder to regain range of movement following TKR in comparison to hip replacements and the range of movement obtained varies. The aim is to obtain 90-degree knee flexion post-operatively (70 degrees minimum). Patients will normally have walking aids (crutches or sticks) which they can gradually discard as they feel able.

If knee movement is progressively *decreasing* or patients are having increasing difficulty with activities of daily living, referral for therapy is indicated.

Signs of inflammation should be heeded with reduced activity, ice and medication.

Arthroscopy

Diagnostic arthroscopy, washouts. These procedures may result in pain and swelling which may take up to 2 weeks to settle. Patients are normally seen by a physiotherapist and advised on a home exercise programme. Outpatient physiotherapy may be arranged, depending on the pathology found and the level of disability the patient is experiencing.

Arthroscopic meniscectomy. These patients may follow a similar routine to above.

Anterior cruciate ligament reconstruction

There are numerous post-operative regimes which are used, therefore check local protocols. These can vary from immobilization in casts for 6 weeks (now rare) to immediate mobilization and weight bearing as tolerated. Comprehensive rehabilitation is normally instigated via the hospital orthopaedic or physiotherapy department and may continue for 6 months.

Examples of return to functional activities for those with immediate mobilization and weight-bearing programme following reconstruction using the hamstring or middle third of the patella tendon are approximately:

- Sedentary work – 3–4 weeks.
- Driving – 4–6 weeks.
- Manual work – 8 weeks.

FOOT AND ANKLE

General advice for people with foot and ankle problems

- With recent onset ankle injuries advise rest in elevation with ice and compression. Address problems with gait (see point below). If not improving (within days), refer to chartered physiotherapist.
- If unable to weight bear comfortably, and the patient has a significantly altered gait pattern, use sticks and crutches to aim to normalize gait pattern. Use stick in *opposite* hand to side with the problem.
- Encourage movement without loading or twisting stresses (i.e. non-weight-bearing exercises, progress to exercises in sitting and then to standing).
- Try 'contrast baths'– using alternate hot and cold immersions for pain relief (30 seconds to 1 minute in each for up to 10 minutes).
- Wear good supportive and appropriate footwear (particularly if running/sports). Be aware that high heel tabs can aggravate (or cause) some Achilles tendonitis problems. If necessary, advise patients to cut the heel tabs down.
- Do not return to running or sports involving running unless the patient can go up onto tiptoe on symptomatic side and hop on that leg without symptoms. In addition they may need to be able to change direction at speed, therefore they should practise figure-of-eight running with direction changes etc., and general training warm-up before returning to their sport.

Ankle exercises

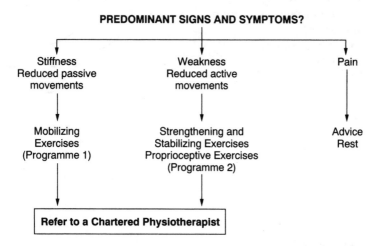

PREDOMINANT SIGNS AND SYMPTOMS?

Stiffness
Reduced passive
movements

Weakness
Reduced active
movements

Pain

↓

↓

↓

Mobilizing
Exercises
(Programme 1)

Strengthening and
Stabilizing Exercises
Proprioceptive Exercises
(Programme 2)

Advice
Rest

Refer to a Chartered Physiotherapist

Foot exercises

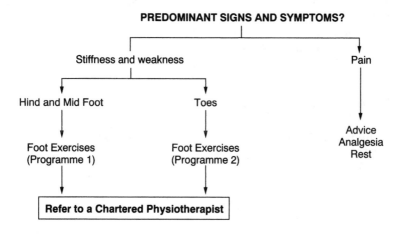

PREDOMINANT SIGNS AND SYMPTOMS?

Stiffness and weakness

Pain

Hind and Mid Foot

Toes

Advice
Analgesia
Rest

Foot Exercises
(Programme 1)

Foot Exercises
(Programme 2)

Refer to a Chartered Physiotherapist

Mobilizing exercises for the ankle

Ankle exercises programme 1

For patients with predominant signs and symptoms of *ankle stiffness*.

Start weight-bearing exercises as soon as possible as they are more functionally relevant.

Non-weight-bearing exercises
Ankle plantarflexion
Sit with leg supported (in elevation
if swelling present)
Heel off end of bed/pillow
Point toes and foot down
Repeat 10 times

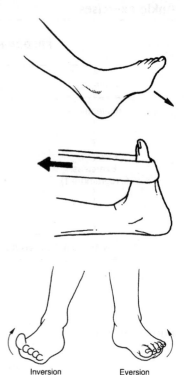

Ankle dorsiflexion
Sit with leg supported (in elevation
if swelling present)
Heel off end of bed/pillow
Pull toes up towards knee
Use a scarf/belt to give extra pressure
Repeat 10 times

Ankle inversion and eversion
Sit with leg supported (in elevation if
swelling present)
Heel off end of bed/pillow
Turn soles of feet
1. to face each other
2. away from each other
Keep knees/legs still
Repeat 10 times each movement

Inversion   Eversion

Progress to

**Ankle plantarflexion and dorsiflexion
in sitting**
Sitting with feet on floor
Raise heels
Then raise toes
Alternate feet (like walking pattern)
Repeat 10 times each direction

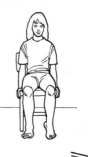

Weight-bearing exercises
Ankle dorsiflexion: calf stretches
Stand with affected leg back in a
walking position
Lean forwards (can use chair/wall
for support)
Keep the back leg straight, heel on ground
Feel the stretch in calf
Hold 20 seconds, repeat 5 times

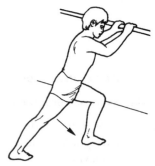

Ankle dorsiflexion: small dips
Stand sideways on a step/large book
Keep foot flat
Bend knee (so it is moving over 2nd toe)
Hold on for balance if necessary (to begin with)
Repeat 10 times
Progress by standing facing forwards

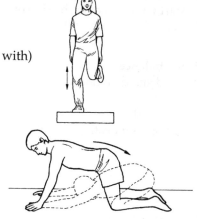

Ankle plantarflexion: kneeling
Kneel on all fours
Gently sit back towards heels
Repeat 5–10 times

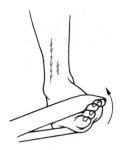

Strengthening and stabilizing exercises for the ankle

Ankle exercises programme 2

For patients with signs and symptoms of ankle *weakness* and feelings of *instability*.
   The muscles that commonly require strengthening are the ankle evertors and plantarflexors. Proprioceptive retraining is also important.

Ankle evertors
Sitting with foot dangling
Lift foot up with sole of foot
facing outwards
Do not let knee move
Then lower it down slowly
Repeat 20–30 times

Progress by
1. placing a weight on foot
2. using elastic cord/rubber banding
3. can use other foot as resistance (cross feet)

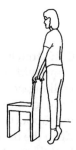

Ankle plantarflexors
Standing on both legs, weight equal on both feet
Go up onto tiptoe
Rest down
Try and make symptomatic side work at least 50%
Repeat 20 times

Progress by
1. when on tiptoe, step to the side with the other leg
2. tiptoe walk

3. do exercise standing on one leg
4. start with heel over the side of step to get stretch
5. hop

Static balance
Try and stand on one leg
Eyes open
Eyes closed
Progress by repeating but on tiptoe

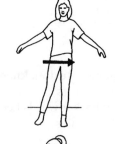

Dynamic balance
Stand on one leg
Keep body upright
Bend knee slowly, making sure knee is
moving over 2nd toe
Keep heel on the ground
Start with small dips and increase gradually
(without pain)
Repeat 10–15 times, once a day minimum

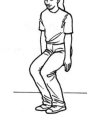

Progress by
1. hopping side to side (keeping alignment)
2. hopping forwards and back (keeping alignment)

Foot exercises programme 1

For patients with signs and symptoms relating to the *hindfoot and midfoot*.

Intrinsics
Sit with foot on floor
Keep toes straight
Draw foot up as if it has become 'shortened'
Hold for 5 seconds
Repeat 20 times
(can do this with shoes on, and in standing)

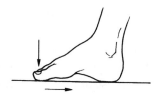

Calf stretches
Stand with affected leg back in a
walking position
Lean forwards (can use chair/wall
for support)
Keep the back leg straight, heel on ground
Feel the stretch in calf

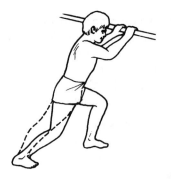

Hold 20 seconds
Repeat 5 times
Repeat with same position as above,
but bend the back leg
Keep heel on ground
Feel stretch in calf, possibly nearer
Achilles tendon
Hold for 20 seconds
Repeat 5 times

Tiptoe standing
Push up onto toes
Lower slowly
Progress to doing without support
(balance or some weight)
Then progress to doing on one leg
Repeat 20 times

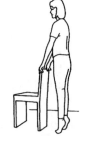

Dynamic alignment work in standing
Stand with feet hip-width apart
Keep body upright
Bend knees fairly slowly, making sure
knees are moving over 2nd toe. When
looking down inside knees, should see
big toes
Keep heels on the ground
Start with small dips and increase
gradually (without pain)
Repeat 10–15 times, once a day
minimum
Progress further by doing on one leg,
maintaining balance

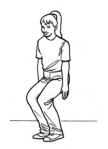

Foot exercises programme 2

For patients with signs and symptoms in the *forefoot (toes)*.

Toe flexion
Sit with a strip of paper towel or a thin
towel under foot
Curl toes up to crumple towel
under foot
Repeat 10 times

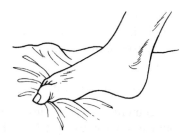

Toe extension
Sit with foot flat on ground
Raise heel, keeping toes on the ground
Get bend at metatarsal-phalangeal joint
Repeat 5 to 10 times

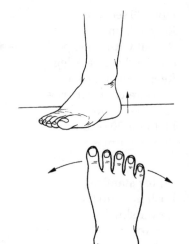

Toe abduction
This is difficult to do but does improve
with practice
Sit with foot on ground
Spread toes apart and together
Try and take big toe out to the side
(towards the other foot)
Repeat 5 to 10 times (or until fatigued)

Post-operative management and advice

Patients are advised to:

- Elevate the foot/feet until the wounds are healed.
- Try and wear spacious and supportive footwear. Gradually build up their tolerance to wearing shoes again, starting with a few minutes each day.

Bunion surgery (bunionectomy, Keller's, Mitchell's osteotomy)

Patients are normally mobilized, heel-walking with crutches. Bunionectomy and Keller's operations are done as day cases with osteotomy patients in hospital for up to 2 days. They are discharged when safe for functional requirements.

Thermoplastic splints or strapping are maintained for 8 weeks. During this time patients gradually increase their walking ability, discarding walking aids as able. It may be a further 8 weeks until a shoe can be worn at all, and 6 months for full recovery.

No specific physiotherapy or exercise programme is implemented.

Fusion of toes

The fusion may be held by a pin for 6–8 weeks. This is removed in the outpatient clinic. The post-operative management is similar in format to bunion surgery (see above).

Achilles tendon rupture

Management of this varies (conservative versus surgical repair and early mobilization versus cast immobilization in both cases). Rehabilitation will normally be instigated according to local instructions. Patients normally need help to regain propulsive and proprioceptive function of the lower limb.

APPENDIX 11.1

Heat

Heat is used for pain-relief, reducing muscle spasm, and increasing joint and/or soft tissue extensibility. It can also encourage the healing of injuries or in mild or chronic inflammation.

It can be given satisfactorily using:

- hot water bottles
- wheat bags (heated in the microwave and normally give heat for approximately 20 min)
- warm shower
- warm bath
- soaking hands/feet in warm water. Using rubber gloves on hands will enable warmer water to be used for this area, without giving skin discomfort
- warm swimming pool, jacuzzi
- electrical heat pads.

The old-fashioned infra-red lamp is now rarely used and not recommended. Heat should not be used on:

- acutely inflamed areas, e.g. hot joints, skin which has had radiotherapy or chemical irritants, acute dermatitis or eczema
- areas with an absence of or poor thermal sensation
- areas with ischaemia, which may not allow an adequate vasodilatory response (e.g. arteriosclerosis, Buerger's disease)

Patients with cardiovascular deficiencies or problems with heat-regulating mechanisms may be at risk if totally immersed in warm water.

Contrast baths

This involves immersion in alternate hot (40–45°C) and cold water (from tap) baths. It is useful for limb extremity problems. The limb part is first immersed in the hot bath for 3–4 minutes, and then placed in the cold bath for 1 minute. This cycle is repeated 3–4 times so that the process may last 15–20 minutes.

Cold

Cold is used for reducing pain and muscle spasm. It gives a strong sensory input which can give effective pain relief. It is beneficial in recent trauma in reducing bleeding and rate of swelling.

It can be applied in various different ways:

- *Ice pack*. Crushed ice or frozen peas (small particles make it more malleable) can be made into a pack. The ice can be wrapped in a wet towel and placed on a piece of paper towel over the skin. This does result in a wet mess, but it is effective in delivering cold to the tissues. If the ice or peas are wrapped or contained in plastic, a damp towel should still be placed over the skin. This precaution reduces the risk of an ice burn (a thin layer of oil on the skin will also reduce this risk). In addition, advise patients not to rest the weight of their body or body part on an ice pack (e.g. lying with leg resting on an ice pack under the calf).

- *Ice massage.* Using an ice cube or an ice 'lollipop'. The 'lollipop' is made from water placed in a plastic cup with a stick in it and put in the freezer. The ice blocks are initially wetted and then rubbed over the painful areas in slow circular movements. The patient feels cold, burning to aching, and then a numbness which may take 5–10 minutes to achieve.

- *Ice baths.* This uses a mixture of flaked ice and cold tap water in a container or sink. The limb extremities can be placed into the iced water. The temperature can be changed by altering the proportions of ice to water. Temperatures of about 16–18°C can usually be tolerated for up to 20 minutes.

- *Ice towels.* This involves dipping a terry-towel in a mixture of crushed ice and water, then wringing it out and wrapping it around the problem area for 2–3 minutes before replacing it with a new towel. This tends to be comfortable and does allow the patient to move with the towel on, but one gets very cold hands.

- *Commercially available cold packs (kept in the freezer).* These still should be applied with a wet towel over the skin. They are convenient but may not be as effective in delivering cold to the tissues.

There is the danger of tissue injury – an ice 'burn'. This can occasionally be seen on normal tissues as tenderness and an erythema of the skin, which can appear several hours after the application of ice. In more severe forms, there is fatty necrosis and bruising can accompany the above symptoms and may last for up to 3 weeks.

Caution is advised in the application of ice on areas with local autonomic pain or temperature disturbances.

Ice therapy may not be suitable for patients with medical conditions which will increase cold sensitivity such as Raynaud's phenomenon, Buerger's disease, cryoglobinaemia and cold urticaria.

Care should be taken cooling large areas of the body in patients with hypertension and cardiac disease.

APPENDIX 11.2

Patients requiring help with adaptations at home, work or with hobbies can be referred to the local occupational therapy services (community or hospital, depending on the nature of their problem and recent management).

The Disabled Living Centres Council (DLCC) lists Disabled Living Centres around the UK. Patients can seek help without referral and can try many useful adaptations for home, work and leisure. This can be from simple long-handled cutlery to driving adaptations. Go to www.dlcc.org.uk or telephone 0161 8341044.

Further reading

Clinical Standards Advisory Group 1994 Back pain. HMSO, London

McKenzie R 1983 Treat your own neck. Spinal Publications Ltd., New Zealand

McKenzie R 1985 Treat your own back. Spinal Publications Ltd., New Zealand

Burton A K, Waddell G, Tillotson K M, Summerton N 1999 Information and advice to patients with back pain can have a positive effect: a randomized controlled trial of a novel educational booklet in primary care. Spine 24(23): 2484–2491

Occupational Health Guidelines for the management of low back pain at work at www.facoccmed.ac.uk

Chapter 12

Case histories
William Hamilton

BACKGROUND

These cases have been structured in a short answer format. We have placed them in a fictitious practice with three partners, and a GP registrar.[1] Our suggested answers follow each group of three cases.

CASE HISTORIES

1 Routine appointment

Doreen is 45 years old and works as a cook in the local school. She describes tingling and numbness in both hands, particularly the palms and first three digits. The problem has slowly got worse over the last year, and is most troublesome at night.

What physical signs would you look for?
What other conditions may she have to make your suspected condition more likely?
What treatments can you offer?

2 Emergency slot

Susan, aged 37, developed rheumatoid arthritis as a young woman. Most of her joints have been badly damaged and she is unable to work. Since last night she has been unable to extend her ring and little fingers. It happened quite suddenly as she was drawing her curtains before bed.

What is the likely diagnosis?
Should she be referred?

---

1. For those outside the UK, general practitioner (GP) registrars are doctors who intend to become GPs, and are working in a 3-year programme of appropriate medical posts. This includes 1 year attached to an approved practice. They are much brighter than the GPs in the practice, but this is balanced by the unmeasurable wisdom and experience of the established GPs. Thus both parties learn from each other.

3 Routine appointment

James, now 52, played good-quality club rugby for many years. He only coaches the youth team now, as 'the youngsters seem to have got faster'. For several months he has had pain and swelling of the right knee lasting for 2–3 days after each coaching session. He is tender on the joint line medially, but has a full range of movements.

Is an X-ray likely to help?
What treatments can you offer?

ANSWERS

1 Doreen

This sounds like carpal tunnel syndrome. You will want to look for signs of median nerve dysfunction, including inspecting for wasting of the thenar eminence. You may find reduced power in thumb and finger flexion, and reduced sensation over the radial 3½ digits on the palmar side.

It would be worth considering hypothyroidism. Pregnancy is unlikely but not impossible, and carpal tunnel may follow rheumatoid arthritis. Rarities like amyloidosis appear much more often in examinations and textbooks than in real life.

Resting the wrist may help, but may be difficult to organize around her job. Analgesia, and night splintage may help. Injection may be beneficial. Referral may be required if these fail.

2 Susan

She has ruptured her extensor tendons, presumably when drawing the curtains.

Not only should she be referred, but urgent referral is necessary, as early repair is much more likely to be successful than delayed repair.

3 James

The decision about James's X-ray is based on whether it is likely to establish a diagnosis, and thus likely to alter treatment. Early osteoarthritis is the likeliest diagnosis clinically, and the X-ray is unlikely to reveal anything surprising. Indeed, many people without symptoms have osteoarthritis radiologically. This could be discussed with James, and an X-ray deferred if he agrees. Having said that, some patients will want their diagnosis 'proven', and an X-ray for that reason would be reasonable, even though this is contrary to the 1998 College of Radiologists' Guidelines. These recommend X-rays only with locking (looking for loose bodies) or if surgery is being considered.

He may well benefit from simple analgesia and a discussion of the prognosis. Physiotherapy and intra-articular steroid injection can help. Some patients find help from arthroscopic washouts but these are used selectively in recurrent cases.

CASE HISTORIES

4 Emergency slot

Darren, aged 19, is the star of the local football team. A heavy tackle on Saturday injured his knee. He struggled on, but had to stop playing after a further 10 minutes, as the knee was too sore. It is still painful on all movements, and is especially tender over the medial collateral ligament. He asks, 'Have I done my cartilage?'

How will you examine him to answer his question?
What treatment can you suggest if it is a ligament strain?
Can he play next Saturday?

5 Routine appointment

Eric is a 79-year-old retired accountant. He rarely attends surgery. He has had 'miserable' back pain for 2 weeks, centred on his lumbar spine, with no radiation to his legs. Simple painkillers have helped a little, but he has hardly slept for the past 3 nights. He is in obvious pain, but allows you to examine his back. Straight leg raising is restricted at 70 degrees because of back pain.

What are the red flags for back pain? How many does Eric have?
What investigations should you do?
Should he be referred, and if so, how urgently?

6 Routine appointment

Rebecca is a secretary for a legal firm, and types lengthy reports for them. She is 29 years old. She has been suffering from pain in the left forearm for 3 weeks now, which she is sure is related to her work. She is tender over the lateral epicondyle.

Assuming she has lateral epicondylitis, or tennis elbow, what treatments could you offer?
Are there any modifications at work which may help?

ANSWERS

4 Darren

Before you examine him, it is worth asking a bit more about the tackle. Did he twist the knee? Was the blow from a particular direction? By doing this you can often gain clues as to the expected injury. However, like all footballers, he wants to know if the problem is his cartilage. You will look for a joint effusion with joint line tenderness. A positive McMurray's test (see page 65), with or without a clunk, will make the diagnosis. A minor flexion deformity with a springy block to extension suggests a large cartilage tear. Doubt over the result of these tests may mean referral is required.

For a strain of the medial collateral ligament, the main treatments are support and analgesia. Rest until the fibres have healed is wise.

Can he play next Saturday? Probably not, as his ligament damage is not minor, given that he is painful to all movements 3 days after the injury, and the ligament is tender. A second injury to this ligament may be much worse.

5 Eric

The red flags are listed on page 42. He has two certain ones (age >55; constant, progressive, non-mechanical back pain). His restricted straight leg raising does not strictly qualify, but is worrisome. The fact that he rarely attends surgery suggests he regards this problem as significant.

Urgent investigation with lumbar spine X-rays and a full blood count with an ESR – as a minimum – are required. If examination suggests a primary cancer such as lung, colorectal or prostate, then these will also need rapid investigation.

Referral partly depends on how well you can control Eric's pain. It is reasonable to offer strong analgesia while organizing rapid investigation. Any symptom or sign suggesting spinal cord damage needs urgent referral, as immediate treatment may prevent paraplegia.

6 Rebecca

Lateral epicondylitis may respond to rest, analgesia with NSAIDs, or steroid injection. Occasionally referral may be needed if these measures fail.

It may well be worth asking about her keyboard and level of support for the wrist and arms. Occupational therapy advice is often very helpful, particularly in reminding employers of their obligation to offer a healthy workplace!

CASE HISTORIES

Wednesday morning surgery is a joint one with GP and registrar.

7 Routine appointment

Selwyn is the 55-year-old director of a wine importing company. He has noticed a thickening in his right palm, and recently his ring finger will not fully extend. The registrar has no difficulty in diagnosing a Dupuytren's contracture.

Are there any primary care treatments for this condition?
Could his occupation be relevant?
If he has surgery, is he likely to need physiotherapy?

8 Routine appointment

Emily is 19 and a student. She has noticed a small, pea-sized lump on the back of her hand. It is not painful. The registrar, now thinking orthopaedics diagnosis is easy, correctly identifies it as a ganglion. However, Emily's question is, 'Can you remove it today? All my friends say how ugly it is.'

How should the registrar respond?

9 Emergency slot

A local builder, Robert, aged 48, limps into your room in obvious pain. He was using a crowbar to break up concrete, missed and plunged the crowbar onto his big toe. There is a large haematoma under his nail.

How can you help him?
Does he need an X-ray?

ANSWERS

7 Selwyn

Are there any primary care treatments for this condition? The short answer is no. So is the long answer.

Dupuytren's contracture is more common in alcoholics, those who use vibrating tools, those on anticonvulsants and Icelanders. It may be worth asking Selwyn how much alcohol he takes.

Post-operative physiotherapy may be helpful: to build on the increase in finger extension that should follow surgery, and to ensure that flexion remains good.

8 Emily

Effectively there are two issues here: the 'correct' management of a ganglion, and how to deal with an unexpected – even inappropriate – request. Dealing with the first: you will want to explain the natural history (about 40% will disappear after a decade) and the treatment possibilities (aspiration with a wide-bore needle, or for big, painful ganglia, excision). The 'inappropriateness' issue is best addressed by putting yourself in her shoes. Who else could she come to for advice about a lump on her hand? Maybe her request for instant cure was pointed, but this gives you an opportunity to discuss health-seeking behaviour, which all GPs are expected to be good at!

9 Robert

The pressure of blood collected under the toenail can be reduced by puncturing the toenail with a heated wire. This can bring considerable relief.

An X-ray is only needed if you think there may be a fracture spreading into the distal interphalangeal joint. So, in the large majority an X-ray will not be needed. There are no significant adverse consequences of 'missing' a small fracture of the distal phalanx.

CASE HISTORIES

10 Home visit

Arthur is 88 years old and lives with his wife of the same age. They have no children. They live together in a small cottage. Arthur has had increasing pain in both hips for many years. He is just able to walk around with a stick, but now cannot climb the stairs to their bedroom. Although analgesia initially helped, codeine-based painkillers make him constipated. He has home support, but he and his wife think they will be unable to stay at home much longer.

Assuming he has osteoarthritis, are there any simple measures you can offer?
How realistic is it to refer him for hip replacement?

11 Routine appointment

Simon, aged 28, made a great rugby tackle 6 months ago but dislocated his shoulder doing so. The same shoulder has dislocated a further three times since, the most recent occasion being 3 nights ago in bed. All of the dislocations have been anterior. He had to attend his local accident and emergency department each time for sedation and relocation of the joint. He asks you if anything can be done to prevent this happening again.

What have you got to offer Simon?
How likely is treatment to be successful?

12 Routine appointment

Sean is 19 years old and had a fantastic holiday with his mates in Kenya 6 months ago. He enjoyed the sun, the sea, and in all likelihood, the local women. A spell of diarrhoea and a urethral discharge were all put down as part of the experience. He now complains of a swollen tender knee. There is an obvious effusion, and the knee is hot.

What diagnoses are you thinking of?
How do you confirm, or refute your diagnoses?
Make a management plan for him.

ANSWERS

10 Arthur

Both Arthur and his wife may benefit from a package of care, not just orthopaedic assessment of Arthur's hip. An occupational therapist may be able to offer advice and support, including various aids for walking, and possibly alterations to the cottage. You, your district nurse or health visitor may be able to help with his constipation. Are there day care facilities that he might wish to attend, allowing his wife some time free of concern about him? Can your local rehabilitation unit help to improve his functioning? Can you find an analgesic that suits?

Hip replacement is feasible even at this age. It may make a dramatic difference to Arthur and his wife. Referral should be discussed with him.

11 Simon

It is time to refer him for surgical stabilization of the shoulder.

Results from surgery are good, with the large majority of patients freed from their problem. This contrasts with surgery for multidirectional instability, associated with a congenitally loose capsule, which is best treated with physiotherapy. Simon should be able to return to rugby after 6 months.

12 Sean

Be careful. We have given you enough clues to make you think of Reiter's syndrome (urethral discharge, gastrointestinal infection, correct timescale). Alternatively, this knee problem may be a response to an injury. However, septic arthritis is a real possibility and a disaster if undiagnosed.

With septic arthritis the patient is usually clearly unwell, and often has a fever. The joint is extremely painful to move, and the effusion tense. With Reiter's syndrome the picture is generally milder. Synovitis, cartilage or ligament damage following trauma is usually suggested by the history. Nonetheless, if you suspect septic arthritis of the knee (or any joint) emergency referral is required. Joint aspiration should be carried out in hospital.

The management plan begins with deciding if septic arthritis is a real possibility: if it is, then refer him. Assuming you have not referred him, the next issue is to organize pain relief. NSAIDs would be the first choice. If there has been no trauma it is likely he has a reactive arthritis such as Reiter's syndrome, or an atypical first presentation of one of the systemic polyarthritides such as rheumatoid arthritis. These will require appropriate investigation and sometimes rheumatological referral.

CASE HISTORIES

13 Emergency slot

Joy is 22 months old. She is the firstborn, after her mother had several miscarriages. Her parents were swinging her up between them in the local park when her arm started hurting. Joy will not move her elbow and holds her arm across her chest. You are able to elicit some tenderness over the radial head.

What is the diagnosis?
Can you help them in your surgery?

14 Routine appointment

Olive is 70 years old and still helps out 3 days a week sorting out donations to a local charity shop. She is getting increasing pain, swelling and stiffness at the base of her right thumb. She asks what you think the diagnosis is, and whether she can continue at work.

What is the likely diagnosis?
Should the joint be X-rayed?
What treatments may help?

15 Routine appointment

Kevin is a hospital porter aged 43. He loves his job, and you remember him from your hospital days. He describes increasing trouble from his heel, with pain so severe that he has had to take time off work. This is his first time off work for many years. He is tender on the bottom of the heel.

What is the likely diagnosis?
Do you X-ray this foot, looking for a calcaneal spur?
What treatments can you offer?

ANSWERS

13 Joy

She has a pulled elbow.

The best treatment for her is to pop the radial head back through the annular ligament as described in the text. Pain relief is usually instant, and your reputation will be enhanced.

14 Olive

It is very likely that this is osteoarthritis of the first metacarpophalangeal joint. It is a common condition and often presents at this age.

It is hard to be dogmatic about this.[2] Issues to consider are your own confidence and experience, and the patient's expectations. Clinical diagnosis is generally easy and little will be lost by deciding against an X-ray.

Treatment includes analgesia, splintage, or a steroid injection. These may well diminish the problem enough for her to continue at work, but she could be referred if the pain continues to be a big problem.

15 Kevin

This is plantar fasciitis. The tenderness is frequently very localized. It is possible his job has contributed to the problem with standing and pushing trolleys along the lengthy corridors.

No. What use is the calcaneal spur (if there is one) in establishing a diagnosis or a prognosis?

Treatment is initially with NSAIDs, plus physiotherapy. Different footwear may help, such as training shoes, or silicone or rubber heel pads. These act to displace the patient's weight from the troublesome part. If these are unhelpful, a long-acting steroid injection may help. Although effective, it is usually very painful.

2. Yes, we know we set the questions, so should have the answers. However, neither orthopaedics nor primary care are black and white, and it would be wrong to pretend that this is so.

CASE HISTORIES

16 Emergency slot

Bethany is 3 years old. Her mother brings her to surgery with the following story. The parents were woken by a thumping noise, and found Bethany on the floor beside her bed. She was upset, but after her parents comforted her she fell asleep again within a quarter of an hour. In the morning her head was rotated 45 degrees to one side, and she was unwilling, or unable, to straighten it.

What do you do?

17 Routine appointment

Jane is a popular local dentist, who is now 52 years old. Over the past few years her neck has given her increasing bother. It is painful, especially after a long session at her dental surgery. She can still move the neck quite well, but towards the extremes of the range of movements it is particularly sore. Simple analgesics help, and a fortnight's break in the south of France helped a lot. Within a few days back at work her pain was back. She asks if you can do anything for her, and whether she should be thinking of early retirement.

Can you do anything for her?
Should she retire?

18 Telephone call

Ian is 38 and a financial expert, with a vast salary. He was logging some trees in the wood by his house. As he bent over to shift a log, he felt a sudden awful pain in his lower back, followed by an 'electric shock' sensation shooting down his right leg. He was unable to get up, but luckily his wife heard his yells for help. With assistance they get him back to the house, and request an urgent home visit at 9.45 a.m. Surgery is due to finish at 11.30.

Do you go? If so, do you attend straight away?
Once you see Ian, what examination do you do?

ANSWERS

16 Bethany

This appears to be a simple torticollis, brought on by the fall from bed. Gentle examination of the head and neck to exclude trauma would be wise, even though the parents are sure to have checked themselves. The vast majority settle without active treatment. If it persists more than a few days, physiotherapy input may be very helpful. A severe torticollis may benefit from referral for inpatient therapy and intensive physiotherapy.

17 Jane

Probably a diagnosis is required first of all. Both you and she will be thinking of cervical spondylosis, and this diagnosis can usually be made without an X-ray. Again, you need to think how X-ray will change your management – generally it will not. Correlation between radiological severity and clinical severity is weak. Jane should be reassured that cervical spondylosis is not always progressive, and in some people symptoms remit after a few years. Some patients benefit from a collar (though this would be very tricky for Jane at work). Physiotherapy and a review of analgesia may well help. Few patients need referral, and even fewer need surgery.

The decision to retire (presumably on medical grounds) is rarely simple. At this stage, when only very simple measures have been tried, it seems premature. She may well benefit from advice from the local occupational health specialists, and may want to consider part-time work.

18 Ian

Most doctors regard severe pain as a fair reason for urgent treatment. Thus your decision whether to go (and how immediately) will depend on your ability to find out how bad his pain now is. The traditional solution of going on the visit and 'offering' the rest of your surgery to the registrar is frowned upon by the educational authorities, but certainly tests if they can cope under pressure!

You will wish to find out if this is an acute disc prolapse or a muscular tear. In favour of a disc prolapse would be the leg pain being worse than the back pain; radiation to the toes and a reduced straight leg raise reproduces the leg pain. The prognosis is worse for disc prolapses, with only half better by 6 weeks. Initially, rest and appropriate analgesia are needed. Physiotherapy is beneficial, and referral at the 6-week point if he is not improving. Earlier rapid referral is indicated if he has uncontrollable pain or limb weakness, or sphincter disturbance.

CASE HISTORIES

19 Routine appointment

Claire is 23 years old and works as a filing clerk in a light engineering company. She was a passenger in a road accident 3 months ago. The vehicle she
was in was hit from behind by a lorry. She went to accident and emergency at
the time, but has not seen you since the accident. She tells you that she has had
pain in her neck since the accident and has been unable to work. She has a
form for her insurance company as she is claiming sickness benefit from them.
She asks you to complete the form for her.

What do you plan to do?

20 Routine appointment

Arthur has been a keen long-distance walker for years. He is surprisingly fit
for his 65 years. Last weekend he was climbing up a steep rocky slope when
his foot slipped. The injury forced his foot upwards rapidly, and was followed
by immediate pain over his Achilles tendon. After a 15 minute break he was
able slowly to return to his car about a mile away. In the 3 days since the
injury, his Achilles tendon has become more swollen and painful.

How can you tell if the tendon is ruptured?
Should you refer him to an orthopaedic surgeon?
What treatment can you offer him?

21 Routine appointment

Edith is a 63-year-old housewife. You rarely see her in surgery. She is suffering
from increasing pain and stiffness in her right shoulder. This has been present
for a month, and there was no obvious precipitant. Almost any movement
is painful, and your examination shows a marked reduction in the range of
movements.

What is the likely diagnosis?
What is the likely prognosis?
Will physiotherapy be helpful?

ANSWERS

19 Claire

Whiplash can last this long, and can prevent work.[3] Certainly there are odd features about this presentation, like why has she not seen you before now, and why has she not requested a sickness certificate? However, you will want to be fair both to her and to the insurance company, by completing the form accurately.

So a short history is required, including detailing how her pain affects leisure activities as well as work; what makes the pain worse or better; what treatment she has had and if there are other injuries or psychological sequelae. An examination of the neck will concentrate on the range of movements and any associated pain.

By doing this, a factual report can be made. You are not the insurance company's secret agent, but equally you will not wish to corroborate possible fraud. By restricting yourself to facts you can steer the correct middle course.

20 Arthur

Thompson's test is the solution. Lie Arthur face down on the examination couch. Squeeze the calf on the affected side and look for plantarflexion of the foot. If the tendon is ruptured almost no movement will occur. Check this against the other side.

If the tendon is not ruptured, treatment can be offered in primary care. With a rupture immediate referral is required. This is especially important now 3 days have passed. If your surgery is far from the orthopaedic centre, cooling the tendon with an ice-pack can be helpful for recent injuries.

Primary care treatment is based on analgesia. Some patients find raising the heel makes the foot more comfortable. Immobilization with plaster of paris is sometimes required for 4 weeks.

21 Edith

This is a frozen shoulder (adhesive capsulitis). Osteoarthritis is unlikely given the short history and restriction of movement.

Most frozen shoulders are better within 3 years, and often less. There is an initial inflammatory phase, followed by stiffness.

Physiotherapy is most helpful in the stiffness phase. It can provoke a worsening of pain in the early stages, when the focus of treatment is on relief of pain and inflammation. This can be by anti-inflammatory medication, or in more severe cases an intra-articular injection of lidocaine (lignocaine).

---

3. If these questions had allowed you to select two out of three cases to answer, we suspect you would have picked the other two. However, primary care and orthopaedics are not like that. Therefore, the tempting answer, 'Ask her to see my partner, Dr Smith, next week – he's good at necks', is not acceptable. Think what choice problems Dr Smith will dump on you the week after.

CASE HISTORIES

22 Routine appointment

Martin attends the surgery frequently with his backache, mostly to collect a prescription for painkillers. The pain is central, and worsened by bending. He has been unable to work for many years (he is aged 43) because of his back pain. He had been a labourer on a building site. Your enthusiastic previous registrar had him assessed by the orthopaedic department a year ago, and they ruled out the prospect of surgery after a full examination. Martin says towards the end of the consultation, 'I'd really love to be better. Have you any bright ideas?'

Well, have you any bright ideas?

23 Routine appointment

Ishmael is 37 years old and has a very successful business in wholesale catering goods. You frequently see his supply van in the town, dropping off deliveries. He attends surgery complaining that his shoulder is sore, particularly when he stretches up to get something from the van. You examine him and he has a clear arc of pain on abduction from about 90 to about 130 degrees. He asks you to draw a diagram showing what is going on in his joint.

Try and draw the diagram for him.
What treatments will you suggest?

24 Routine appointment

Gregory, aged 78, retired years ago. He fervently supports the local football team. Over the last few months he has noticed vague difficulties with walking and balance. He dropped a plastic cup of tea at half-time at a match recently. When you examine him, you find that his muscle power in his legs is reduced and his plantar reflexes are upgoing.

What is the differential diagnosis?
What other questions should you ask him?

ANSWERS

22 Martin

Assuming the orthopaedic assessment last year was thorough, there seems little point in repeating it. Therefore, you can concentrate on other ways of helping him. One possibility is using a rehabilitation team. These are usually a combination of orthopaedic surgeon, a physiotherapist, a pain specialist and a psychologist. The exact make-up of the team varies. The emphasis is not on 'curing' the pain but helping the patient to live with it. They may also have complementary therapies available, such as osteopathy, chiropractic or acupuncture. Thinking more radically, Martin may be interested in retraining to a new trade. There are specialized centres in the UK and elsewhere aimed at retraining people with disabilities.

Finally, the classic GP trick. How about asking Martin if he has any bright ideas himself? Could his question have been a way of introducing a possible treatment he has heard of and wonders what you think?

Of course, many patients with this problem remain incapacitated: however, that is no reason not to try and help.

23 Ishmael

We hope your diagram approximates to the one on page 5. The key feature is that a painful arc is produced by the greater tuberosity of the humerus impinging on the coraco-acromial ligament and the acromion.

Treatment comes in two parts: analgesia with NSAIDs and physiotherapy. If these do not help, an injection into the subacromial region with anaesthetic and steroid is the next step. After 3–6 months, referral may be required, for consideration of surgery.

24 Gregory

This is a worrying picture, with symptoms and signs suggesting an upper motor neurone lesion. Furthermore, his spill with the cup may signify that the nerve supply to the arms is compromised too (we know you did a splendid neurological examination of the arms as well as the legs, and it looks as if you found nothing[4]). Top of the list is cervical myelopathy, but you will want to consider multiple small strokes, tumours, even cord degeneration from vitamin B_{12} deficiency. He qualifies for urgent referral to confirm or exclude cervical stenosis.

It is easy to forget to ask about bowel and bladder function, but they can both be compromised in cervical myelopathy. You should also ask about Lhermitte's phenomenon. This occurs when the neck is flexed or extended and the patient feels a tingling sensation travelling down their limbs or even into their head.

---

4. Of course, you looked for a Hoffman's sign – by flicking the palmar surface of the middle finger and watching if the index finger or thumb moved upwards.

CASE HISTORIES

25 Telephone call from the district nurse

She was visiting to give an elderly blind diabetic patient her insulin, and found the patient's son, Brian, aged 48, stuporose on the floor. There was a strong smell of alcohol. This is no surprise as Brian is well known to the practice for his alcoholism (so much so that he isn't trusted to give his mother her insulin). The district nurse is concerned that Brian may have injured himself, and suggests he may have fractured his neck of femur. You come to the house quickly.

How can you tell if a patient has a fractured neck of femur, especially with no history available?

26 Routine appointment

Adrian, aged 28, is the first patient in afternoon surgery. He has pain localized to a small area on the radial side of his right wrist. It is very troublesome after a game of squash. Rest and painkillers have not helped.

What is the likely diagnosis?
What physical sign do you look for?
What treatments may help?

27 Routine appointment

Lee is 13 years old and accompanied by his mother. He is shy so she tells the story. Every time he walks to school he begins to complain of pain in the right knee. She thought he was trying to get her to drive him there (it is only 500 metres from home to school), but realized something was wrong when he continued to complain at weekends. At times he gets a clicking sensation in the joint.

When you examine him you find a mild effusion, and his quadriceps look wasted when compared with the other side. It is slightly tender on the medial side.
What is the likeliest diagnosis?
Do you refer?

ANSWERS

25 Brian

The crucial thing is adequate inspection. You will have to get Brian in a position where you can see whether one leg is shorter than the other. The shortened leg will also be externally rotated, if it is indeed a fracture. You would expect it to be painful but this may be very difficult to assess in Brian's state. Fractured necks of femur are easy to miss, but even easier to miss if you don't think of the possibility. We do not all have orthopaedic experts as district nurses. If there is any clinical doubt, referral is sensible.[5]

26 Adrian

He probably has de Quervain's tenosynovitis. This is due to inflammation of the abductor pollicis tendon sheath.

Finkelstein's test is diagnostic, but easier to do than describe. Bend the patient's thumb into the palm, and wrap the fingers around it in a sort of fist. Now move the fist in an ulnar direction (away from the site of the pain). This should reproduce pain over the tendon sheath.

Adrian has tried rest, so the next option is to splint the thumb, and offer NSAIDs. A steroid injection avoiding the subcutaneous tissues can be very effective.

27 Lee

This is osteochondritis dissecans, and the diagnosis can be confirmed by X-ray. This is useful to assess whether the fragment of bone has separated from the femoral condyle.

Surgery is reserved for those whose fragment has separated off. This may cause locking of the joint. Otherwise, treatment consists of rest. Therefore, referral is not essential, but may provide additional reassurance.

---

5. By the way, have you diagnosed Brian's stupor? He may be an alcoholic, but that does not mean this is the only possible cause of his coma. Is he toxic from a septic arthritis, which is causing the hip problem too, and not a fracture after all?

CASE HISTORY

28 Child health surveillance appointment

Your health visitor does the bulk of the child health surveillance in the practice. The format for the 8-week check is that she performs a full examination, with all the heights and weights, etc., and you join her in doing the cardiovascular and hip examination and responding to any concerns raised in the earlier part of the check. This time your health visitor greets you with, 'My only concern with Jasmine is that her hips click when I examine them'.

Although you are clearly going to fully examine Jasmine, what is the key test? If your examination is normal what will you do now?

ANSWER

28 Jasmine

The crucial thing to elucidate is whether Jasmine's hip(s) is unstable. The click your health visitor found is not in itself important. Jasmine's hip has been unstable from birth; by this stage fixed displacement is likely to have occurred. The affected leg is a little shorter, it is externally rotated and the thigh creases are asymmetrical. Crucially when the hips are flexed, and abduction attempted, there is reduced abduction on the affected side.

If the examination is normal, you will want to reassure, but may ask Jasmine's parent to bring her to you for re-checking in a few weeks. However, if there is some doubt, earlier reassessment is sensible, with referral to a specialist if doubt remains.

Index

Note: Page references in *italics* indicate illustrations